Series Editor

Prof. Dr. Michael J. Parnham
PLIVA
Research Institute
Prilaz baruna Filipovica 25
10000 Zagreb
Croatia

Medicinal Fatty Acids in Inflammation

Joel M. Kremer

Editor

Springer Basel AG

Editor

Prof. Dr. Joel M. Kremer
Professor of Medicine
Head, Division of Rheumatology
Albany Medical College
Albany, NY 12208
USA

A CIP catalogue record for this book is available from the Library of Congress, Washington D.C., USA

Deutsche Bibliothek Cataloging-in-Publication Data
Medicinal fatty acids in inflammation / ed. by J. Kremer ... Springer Basel AG 1998

(Progress in inflammation research)
ISBN 978-3-0348-9788-4 ISBN 978-3-0348-8825-7 (eBook)
DOI 10.1007/978-3-0348-8825-7

The publisher and editor can give no guarantee for the information on drug dosage and administration contained in this publication. The respective user must check its accuracy by consulting other sources of reference in each individual case.

Originally published by Birkhäuser Verlag in 1998
Softcover reprint of the hardcover 1st edition 1998
Printed on acid-free paper produced from chlorine-free pulp. TCF ∞
Cover design: Markus Etterich, Basel

ISBN 978-3-0348-9788-4

9 8 7 6 5 4 3 2 1

Contents

List of contributors

Andrea Belluzzi, Department of Emergency Medicine, S. Orsola Hospital, Via Massarenti, 9, I-40138 Bologna, Italy; fax: ++39 51 399 914

Philip C. Calder, Institute of Human Nutrition, University of Southampton, Bassett Crescent East, Southampton SO16 7PX, UK

James V. Donadio, Division of Nephrology, Mayo Clinic, 200 First Street SW, Rochester, MN 55905, USA; e-mail: donadio.james@mayo.edu

Piet P. Geusens, Clinical Research Center for Bone and Joint Diseases, Dr L. Willems-Instituut, Limburgs Universitair Centrum, B-3590 Diepenbeek, Belgium; e-mail: geusens@tornado.be

Joseph P. Grande, Division of Anatomic Pathology, Mayo Clinic, 200 First Street SW, Rochester, MN 55905, USA; e-mail: grande.joseph@mayo.edu

David F. Horrobin, Laxdale Research, King's Park House, Laurelhill Business Park, Stirling, Scotland FK7 9JQ

Federico Miglio, Department of Emergency Medicine, S. Orsola Hospital, Via Massarenti, 9, I-40138 Bologna, Italy; fax: ++39 51 399 914

John B. Rodgers, Albany Medical College, A-48, Department of Medicine, 47 New Scotland Avenue, Albany, NY 12208, USA

Vincent A. Ziboh, Department of Dermatology, TB 192, School of Medicine, University of California, Davis, CA 95616, USA

Robert B. Zurier, University of Massachusetts Medical Center, 55 Lake Avenue North, Worcester, MA 01655, USA; e-mail: robert.zurier@banyan.ummed.edu

Preface

This volume of *Progress in Inflammation Research* is a unique compilation of work performed by a wide spectrum of investigators from different medical disciplines. It is fascinating that dietary alterations of fatty acid intake can result in a range of salutory changes in a great variety of medical conditions. Most of the good scientific work which has led to these observations has been performed over just the last two decades. This is of course not a very long time in the context of the history of the human species. Recently performed analysis of fat intake from paleolithic times has indicated that our hunter-gatherer ancestors consumed as much cholesterol as modern Western man, but strikingly less saturated fatty acid and more polyunsaturates, including *n*-3 fatty acids. Wild game has the terrestrial source of *n*-3 incorporated in its fat since browsing animals derive 18:3*n*-3 (alpha-linolenic acid) naturally from leafy plants.

There is, however, little opportunity for modern Western man to get *n*-3 fatty acids from the diet if one does not consume fish. Modern agribusiness provides animal feeds high in *n*-6 fatty acids, mostly derived from linoleic acid (18:2*n*-6) in corn feed. Therefore, grazing animals have no access to alternative fatty acids in either feed or grasses, the latter containing little or none of these potentially beneficial highly polyunsaturated fatty acids. We have, as a species, passed the overwhelming majority of our time evolving with foods containing *n*-3 fatty acids only to have them removed in the last 200 years. Some have speculated that the prevalence of inflammatory diseases has increased during this same time interval as a direct result of the change in our dietary intake of fatty acids. This is a controversial premise which is difficult, if not impossible, to prove. The evidence is circumstantial at best. There are certainly many other dietary and environmental changes which have occurred in the Western World over the same time interval.

However, only the lipid content of the diet is reflected in the basic structure of the cell. The phospholipid component of the lipid bilayer of the plasma membrane is determined by dietary fatty acid intake. Thus diets rich in *n*-3 or *n*-6 fatty acids including gammalinoleic acid (GLA) will result in the incorporation of these fatty acids into the plasma membrane. There they serve as alternative substrates to arichidonate for oxidative pathways leading to eicosanoid production. This is reviewed in several chapters in this volume. In addition, a host of other cellular changes may occur which result in modifications of immune function. The emerging evidence on the mechanisms of these dietarily induced alterations is found elsewhere in this volume.

We have as a species rounded a scientific corner with this new information. Inflammatory diseases must be added to atherosclerosis and malignancy in an expanding listing of medical conditions which can unequivocally be affected by diet. These advances are the natural outgrowth of both a worldwide heightened interest and awareness of nutrition and the increasingly sophisticated scientific techniques, including those of molecular biology, which have been utilized to explore the mechanism of action of dietary alterations in fatty acids.

As in most new developments which lead to a fundamental alteration in the way people view their world, universal acceptance is often slow to come forth. It is sometimes easier to be a skeptic in the face of new information which alters our view of the natural order of things than to give ourselves over to a new world view. Nevertheless, with the passage of time, the validity of new ideas and observations become accepted with resultant behavioral modifications. This will surely be the case with the description of the effects of fatty acids on inflammation which are found in this volume.

Joel M. Kremer
Albany, USA

March, 1998

n-3 Polyunsaturated fatty acids and mononuclear phagocyte function

Philip C. Calder

Institute of Human Nutrition, University of Southampton, Bassett Crescent East, Southampton SO16 7PX, UK

The mononuclear phagocyte

Definitions and characteristics

The macrophage is the major differentiated cell of the mononuclear phagocyte system. This system comprises bone marrow monoblasts and promonocytes, peripheral blood monocytes and tissue macrophages. Macrophages are widely distributed in the body, displaying great structural and functional heterogeneity. The precursors of these cells originate in the bone marrow, from which incompletely differentiated monocytes enter the peripheral blood. Monocytes are 10 to 20 µm in diameter and have well developed Golgi apparatus, numerous lysosomal granules, evenly distributed mitochondria and a single kidney-shaped nucleus; their half life in the bloodstream is relatively short (< 70 h). Once they have settled in a tissue (such as connective tissue, liver, lung or the peritoneal cavity), monocytes mature and become macrophages. Macrophages are larger than monocytes (10 to 80 µm in diameter) and have an oval-shaped nucleus, a cytoplasm containing numerous dense granules, endocytic vesicles, mitochondria and lysosomes and many pseudopodia extending from the cell surface. In contrast to the short half life of monocytes, macrophages remain in tissues for many months, perhaps even years. Often they are named to designate specific locations; for example, in the central nervous system they are called microglia and in the vascular sinusoids of the liver they are called Kupffer cells. Macrophages sometimes stay relatively quiescent as resident cells; these are tissue macrophages that have not encountered foreign materials and have low functional activities. If they encounter foreign materials, such as microorganisms, they differentiate further becoming more active. This process involves multiple phenomena, but there is general agreement in categorising these cells as inflammatory macrophages, which are high in secretory activity but do not possess microbicidal or tumouricidal activity. In comparison, activated macrophages possess high activity in secreting reactive oxygen metabolites (the superoxide radical and hydrogen peroxide) and cytokines, and

Medicinal Fatty Acids in Inflammation, edited by J. Kremer

have microbicidal and tumouricidal activity. Inflammatory macrophages are stimulated by non-specific inflammatory factors, whereas activated macrophages are stimulated by immunologic factors via lymphocyte-derived cytokines; the term elicited is often used to describe inflammatory macrophages. As a result of the different developmental and environmental factors which prevail, macrophages at one site may become morphologically and functionally different from those at other sites.

Functions of mononuclear phagocytes

Mononuclear phagocytes are critical for natural immunity, but also play a part in specific immunity. Macrophages phagocytose foreign particles or injured or dead cells and they secrete enzymes (e.g. elastase, collagenase), reactive oxygen species (superoxide radicals, hydroxyl radicals, hydrogen peroxide), reactive nitrogen species (nitric oxide), prostaglandins, cytokines and growth factors (Tab. 1). These functions are all part of natural immunity. Macrophages can also behave as antigen-presenting cells, displaying foreign antigens on their cell surface for recognition by antigen-specific T lymphocytes. Macrophages are activated by cytokines, which are released from helper T-cells and enable macrophages to perform their phagocytic and degradative functions more effectively than unstimulated cells. Since they possess receptors for antibodies, macrophages also participate in the elimination of foreign antigens by humoral immune responses. The functions of mononuclear phagocytes have been reviewed in detail [1], and the roles of macrophages in immunity against viruses, bacteria, parasites and tumours have been reviewed [2–5]. Because many of the secretory products of macrophages regulate inflammation or directly cause tissue damage, these cells have been implicated as playing a key role in many chronic inflammatory diseases (see [6] for a review).

Table 1 - Functions of mononuclear phagocytes

Phagocytosis	Secretion	Immunoregulation
Bacteria, fungi, parasites, viruses Biological debris Foreign particles Senescent leukocytes and erythrocytes	Enzymes and molecules involved in inflammation and tissue repair Microbiocidal and tumouricidal molecules Cell growth regulating factors	Antigen presentation Regulation of T- and B-cell function Suppressor factors

Dietary fatty acids and immune cell functions

The pathway for synthesis of polyunsaturated fatty acids (PUFAs) is shown in Figure 1. The introduction of a single double bond between carbon atoms 9 and 10 is catalysed by the enzyme Δ^9-desaturase, which is universally present in both plants and animals. This enzyme results in the conversion of stearic acid (18:0) to oleic acid (18:1*n*-9). Plants, unlike animals, can insert additional double bonds into oleic acid between the existing double bond at the 9-position and the methyl terminus of the carbon chain; a Δ^{12}-desaturase converts oleic acid into linoleic acid (18:2*n*-6) while a Δ^{15}-desaturase converts linoleic acid into α-linolenic acid (18:3*n*-3). Using the pathway outlined in Figure 1, animal cells can convert dietary α-linolenic acid into eicosapentaenoic acid (EPA; 20:5*n*-3) and docosahexaenoic acid (DHA; 22:6*n*-3); by a similar series of reactions, dietary linoleic acid is converted via γ-linolenic (18:3*n*-6) and dihomo-γ-linolenic (20:3*n*-6) acids to arachidonic acid (20:4*n*-6). The *n*-9, *n*-6 and *n*-3 families of PUFAs are not metabolically interconvertible in mammals. Many marine plants, especially the unicellular algae in phytoplankton, also carry out chain elongation and further desaturation of α-linolenic acid to yield the long-chain *n*-3 PUFAs EPA and DHA. It is the formation of these long chain *n*-3 PUFAs by marine algae and their transfer through the food chain to fish, that accounts for their abundance in some marine fish oils. Table 2 lists the principal fatty acids found in various oils which have been used experimentally.

Interest in the effects of fatty acids and dietary lipids upon the immune system dates back many years (see [7] for an early review), but this interest has intensified with the elucidation of the roles of eicosanoids derived from arachidonic acid in modulating inflammation and immunity (see [8–11] for reviews) and with the knowledge that the metabolism of arachidonic acid to yield these mediators can

Table 2 - Principal fatty acids in various dietary oils

Oil	Principal fatty acids
Coconut	Medium chain saturated: capric (10:0), lauric (12:0), myrystic (14:0)
Palm	Palmitic (16:0) comprises 50% fatty acids
Olive	Oleic (18:1*n*-9) comprises 55 to 85% fatty acids
Corn	Linoleic (18:2*n*-6) comprises 40 to 65% fatty acids
Sunflower	Linoleic (18:2*n*-6) comprises 50 to 75% fatty acids
Safflower	Linoleic (18:2*n*-6) comprises 70 to 85% fatty acids
Linseed	α-Linolenic (18:3*n*-3) comprises 35 to 65% fatty acids
Fish (e.g. menhaden)	EPA (20:5*n*-3) comprises 10 to 15% fatty acids DHA (22:6*n*-3) comprises 5 to 12% fatty acids

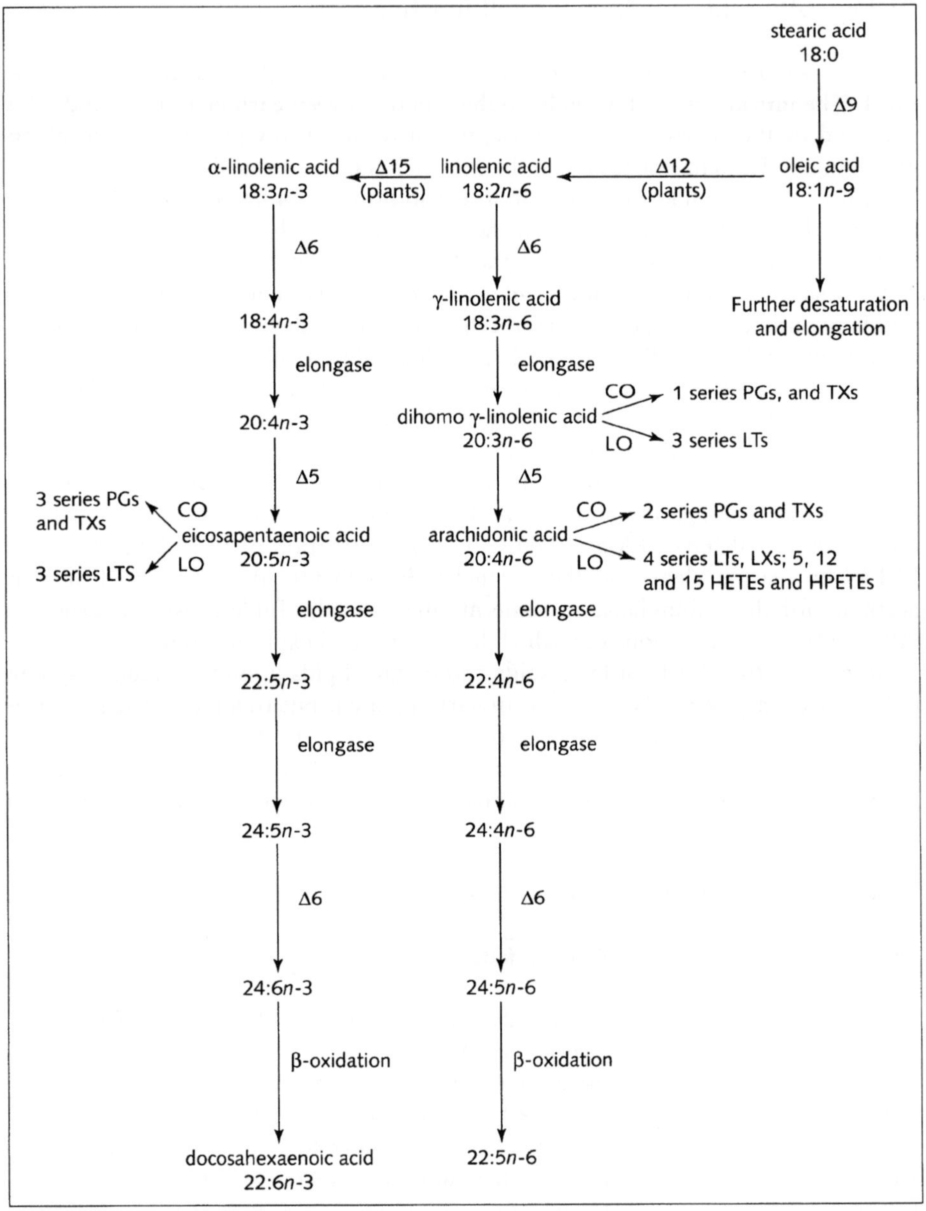

Figure 1
Metabolism of PUFAs. Δ5, 6, 9, 12, 15 indicate desaturase enzymes; CO and LO indicate cyclooxygenase and lipoxygenase enzymes respectively. For further explanations see text.

be inhibited by the long chain n-3 PUFAs found in some marine fish oils (see [11–15] for reviews). Various aspects of lipids and immunity have been reviewed [12–25] and this review will focus on the effects of n-3 PUFAs upon mononuclear phagocyte fatty acid composition, production of eicosanoids, reactive oxygen species, nitric oxide and cytokines and macrophage-mediated phagocytosis and cytolysis.

Effect of n-3 PUFAs on mononuclear phagocyte fatty acid composition

Modification of the total lipid fatty acid profile of macrophages following culture with various fatty acids has been reported [26–28], as has modification of the phospholipid fraction [28–30] and the neutral lipid fraction [30] of the cells. Culture of macrophages with n-3 PUFAs results in replacement of arachidonic acid in phospholipids by the n-3 PUFA provided [27, 30, 31] (Tab. 3).

Dietary lipid modulation also results in significant modification of the fatty acid composition of macrophages isolated from the peritoneal cavity of mice [32–35], rats [36, 37] (Tab. 4) or hamsters [38], or from the lungs of pigs [39] and of monocytes isolated from human peripheral blood [40–42]. Again, one key change is the replacement of arachidonic acid by n-3 PUFAs provided in the diet (Tab. 4).

Table 3 - Fatty acid composition of the phospholipids of murine macrophages cultured with different fatty acids

	Fatty acid (mol/100 mol total fatty acids)				
Addition	**18:2n-6**	**20:4n-6**	**20:5n-3**	**22:5n-3**	**22:6n-3**
Fresh cells	5.2 ± 0.2	15.7 ± 1.1	n.d.	n.d.	1.1 ± 0.3
BSA	4.9 ± 0.4	14.4 ± 1.1	n.d.	n.d.	1.4 ± 0.2
Arachidonic acid	6.4 ± 0.3	27.9 ± 3.1	n.d.	n.d.	0.4 ± 0.1
EPA	3.9 ± 0.4	5.6 ± 0.7	11.8 ± 2.3	1.8 ± 0.4	1.9 ± 0.3
DHA	3.8 ± 0.5	9.7 ± 0.8	1.4 ± 0.5	2.9 ± 0.4	12.7 ± 1.8

Thioglycollate-elicited macrophages obtained from mice fed standard laboratory chow were cultured for 48 h in the presence of 100 μM arachidonic acid, EPA or DHA; the fatty acids were provided to the cells as 1:1 complexes with bovine serum albumin (BSA) and control cells were incubated with BSA. After the culture period macrophage total lipid was extracted and phospholipids isolated; the fatty acid composition of the phospholipid fraction was determined using gas chromatography. Data are mean ± SEM and are taken from ref. [30]; n.d. indicates not detected.

Table 4 - Effect of dietary lipids on the fatty acid composition of the phospholipids of rat macrophages

	Fatty acid (mol/100 mol total fatty acids)				
Diet	**18:2*n*-6**	**20:4*n*-6**	**20:5*n*-3**	**22:5*n*-3**	**22:6*n*-3**
Corn oil	9.5 ± 0.5	14.2 ± 0.8	0.4 ± 0.1	1.8 ± 0.3	1.8 ± 0.3
Corn + linseed oils	10.0 ± 0.4	10.0 ± 0.1	1.2 ± 0.1	3.2 ± 0.1	1.9 ± 0.2
Corn + fish oils	12.2 ± 0.5	9.0 ± 0.4	3.8 ± 0.2	4.1 ± 0.3	3.8 ± 0.2

Rats were fed for 6 weeks on diets containing 65 g/kg of either corn oil, corn + linseed oils or corn + fish oils. Resident peritoneal macrophages were prepared, total lipid was extracted and phospholipids isolated; the fatty acid composition of the phospholipid fraction was determined using gas chromatography. Data are mean ± SEM and are taken from ref. [35].

Effect of *n*-3 PUFAs on eicosanoid production by mononuclear phagocytes

Eicosanoids are a family of oxygenated derivatives of dihomo-γ-linolenic, arachidonic and eicosapentaenoic acids. Eicosanoids include prostaglandins (PGs), thromboxanes (TXs), leukotrienes (LTs), lipoxins (LXs), hydroperoxyeicosatetraenoic acids (HPETEs) and hydroxyeicosatetraenoic acids (HETEs). In most conditions the principal precursor for these compounds is arachidonic acid (Fig. 1). Eicosanoids usually have a short half-life and act locally on the cell from which they are produced. Their production is initiated by particular stimuli and, once produced, they themselves are able to modify the response to the stimulus. PGs are involved in modulating the intensity and duration of inflammatory and immune responses; PGE_2 has a number of pro-inflammatory effects including induction of fever and erythema, increasing vascular permeability and vasodilation and enhancing pain and oedema caused by other agents such as bradykinin and histamine. In chronic inflammatory conditions increased rates of PGE_2 production are observed, and elevated PGE_2 production has been observed in patients suffering from infections, burns, sepsis and other traumas. It appears that each of the lipoxygenase enzymes has a particular cellular distribution: 5-lipoxygenase is found in mast cells, monocytes, macrophages and granulocytes, 12-lipoxygenase is found in platelets and some epithelial cells and 15-lipoxygenase is found in young myeloid cells and some epithelial cells.

The *n*-3 PUFAs, EPA and DHA competitively inhibit the oxygenation of arachidonic acid by cyclooxygenase. In addition, EPA (but not DHA) is able to act as a substrate for both cyclooxygenase and 5-lipoxygenase (Fig. 1). Since ingestion of *n*-3 PUFAs results in decreased membrane arachidonic acid levels (see Tab. 4),

Table 5 - Effect of dietary lipids on the production of arachidonic acid-derived eicosanoids by murine peritoneal macrophages.

	Eicosanoid (ng/ml)		
Diet	**PGE_2**	**6-keto-$PGF_{1\alpha}$**	**TXB_2**
Low fat	73 ± 7	0.7 ± 0.1	0.6 ± 0.1
Coconut oil	52 ± 12	0.7 ± 0.1	0.5 ± 0.2
Safflower oil	60 ± 9	0.8 ± 0.1	0.8 ± 0.1
Fish oil	18 ± 2	0.2 ± 0.1	0.3 ± 0.1

Mice were fed on a low fat (25 g/kg corn oil) diet or on diets containing 200 g/kg of either hydrogenated coconut oil, safflower oil or fish oil. Thioglycollate-elicited peritoneal macrophages were prepared and cultured with bacterial lipopolysaccharide (LPS) (10 µg/ml) for 24 h. The medium was collected and eicosanoid concentrations were measured by ELISA. Data are mean ± SEM and are taken from ref. [43].

there is a concomitant decrease in the capacity of monocytes and macrophages to synthesise eicosanoids from arachidonic acid [32, 33, 36, 39–41, 43–45] (Tab. 5). The suppression in the production of arachidonic acid-derived eicosanoids is mirrored by an elevation in the production of EPA-derived eicosanoids [46], such as the 3-series PGs and TXs and the 5-series LTs. The eicosanoids produced from EPA are often less biologically potent than the analogues synthesised from arachidonic acid.

Effects of *n*-3 PUFAs on production of reactive oxygen species and nitric oxide by macrophages

Production of reactive oxygen species and nitric oxide

The enzymes which result in the synthesis of superoxide, hydrogen peroxide and nitric oxide are regulated by eicosanoids, cytokines and protein kinase C. Since *n*-3 PUFAs affect the production of eicosanoids (see above) and cytokines (see below) and might modulate protein kinase C activity (see [15, 21] for references), they might affect the production of reactive oxygen species and nitric oxide by macrophages and so regulate the cytotoxic activities of these cells. However, investigations of the effects of diets rich in *n*-3 PUFAs upon the production of hydrogen peroxide, superoxide and nitric oxide have yielded contradictory results (see Tab. 6 for references). Studies have reported that production of these mediators is

Table 6 - Summary of studies investigating the effects of dietary n-3 *PUFAs on production of reactive oxygen species or nitric oxide and on phagocytosis by mononuclear phagocytes*

Species	Details of diets used	Cell type	*Ex vivo* stimulus	Observations	Ref.
Human	3.6 g EPA + 2.4 g DHA per day; 6 weeks	Blood monocyte	Zymosan	Superoxide production decreased	47
Human	3.8 g EPA or 3.8 g DHA or 3.8 g corn oil per day; 7 weeks	Blood monocyte	*Eschericia coli*	Respiratory burst unaffected Phagocytosis of unopsonised or opsonised bacteria unaffected Binding of opsonised bacteria by monocytes increased with EPA	42
Rat	80 g/kg coconut, olive, peanut or fish oil; 6 weeks	Resident peritoneal macrophage	LPS	Nitric oxide production: fish < peanut < olive < coconut	48
			PMA	Superoxide and hydrogen peroxide production: fish < peanut < olive < coconut	
Rat	Chow or 150 g/kg fish oil; 6 weeks	Resident peritoneal macrophage	LPS	Nitric oxide production lower with fish oil	49
Rat	Control diet (linoleic acid rich) or 100 g/kg linseed or 62 g/kg defatted linseed; 8 weeks	Resident peritoneal macrophage	PMA	Superoxide production lower with linseed	50
			Listeria monocytogenes	Superoxide production, nitric oxide production and phagocytosis unaffected by diet	
Mouse	100 g/kg safflower or fish oil; 4 weeks	Thioglycollate-elicited peritoneal macrophage	Zymosan	Hydrogen peroxide production lower with fish oil	51
			PMA	Hydrogen peroxide production unaffected by diet	
			Sheep erythrocytes	Phagocytosis unaffected by diet	
			Yeast	Phagocytosis unaffected by diet	

Table 6 (continued)

Species	Details of diets used	Cell type	*Ex vivo* stimulus	Observations	Ref.
Mouse	50 g/kg corn oil + 50 g/kg fish oil or 100 g/kg palm or fish oil; 6 to 15 weeks	Thioglycollate-elicited peritoneal macrophage	IFN-γ	Nitric oxide production higher with fish oil	52
Mouse	Dams fed 100 g/kg olive, safflower, linseed or fish oil; 20 weeks	Thioglycollate-elicited peritoneal macrophage	PMA	Superoxide production higher with fish or linseed oil than with olive or safflower oil	53
Mouse	100 g/kg safflower, linseed or fish oil; 3 weeks	Thioglycollate-elicited peritoneal macrophage	IFN-γ + LPS	Nitric oxide production unaffected by diet	54
Mouse	Low fat (25 g/kg corn oil) or 200 g/kg coconut, olive, safflower or fish oil; 8 weeks	Thioglycollate-elicited peritoneal macrophage	LPS	Nitric oxide production: low fat < olive, safflower, fish, coconut < safflower	43
			PMA	Hydrogen peroxide production higher with fish oil Superoxide production unaffected by diet	
			Zymosan	Hydrogen peroxide production higher with fish oil	
Rat	90 g/kg safflower or fish oil; 12 days	Alveolar macrophage	IFN-γ + LPS	Nitric oxide production higher with fish oil	55
Rabbit	Control diet or control diet + 5 g safflower or fish oil/kg body weight per day by gastric tube; 1 week	Alveolar macrophage	Zymosan	Superoxide production lower with fish oil	56

Table 6 (continued)

Species	Details of diets used	Cell type	*Ex vivo* stimulus	Observations	Ref.
Pig	Standard diet or 105 g/kg corn, linseed or fish oil or 1:1 mixture of corn-linseed or corn-fish oils; 4 weeks	Alveolar macrophage	LPS	Nitric oxide production higher with corn or fish oil or corn-linseed oil mix	57
			Latex beads	No effect on phagocytosis	
Mouse	Low fat (30 g/kg corn oil) or 200g/kg corn or fish oil; 4 weeks	Kupffer	*Salmonella typhimurium*	Phagocytosis lower with fish oil in uninfected animals; Phagocytosis unaffected by diet if animals previously infected with *Salmonella typhimurium*	58
				Number of cells involved in oxidative burst unaffected by diet (but increased by infection)	
				Oxidative burst lower with fish oil than low fat diet in uninfected animals	

PMA indicates phorbol myristyl acetate; IFN-γ indicates interferon-γ enhanced, diminished or not affected following fish oil feeding to laboratory animals (see Tab. 6 for references). The reasons for such significantly different experimental observations might include the different species of origin of the cells studied, the anatomical site of origin of the cells, the state of cellular differentiation, the state of activation of the cell, the stimulus used to elicit mediator production, the nature of the culture conditions used (presence or absence of serum, serum source, time of culture etc.), the level of *n*-3 PUFAs in the diet, the duration of feeding, the level of antioxidants in the diet and so on. In a recent study, thioglycollate-elicited peritoneal macrophages from mice fed 200 g/kg fish oil for 8 weeks produced more hydrogen peroxide in response to stimulation by PMA or zymosan than macrophages from mice fed a low fat diet [43]; production of superoxide from these cells also tended to be elevated. Furthermore, macrophages from the fish oil-fed mice produced more nitric oxide in response to stimulation with LPS than those from mice fed the low fat diet [43]. Since superoxide, hydrogen peroxide and nitric oxide are important macrophage-derived cytotoxic agents these observations suggest that dietary fish oil could affect the killing of microbial or tumour cells by macrophages.

Effects of *n*-3 PUFAs on macrophage-mediated phagocytosis

It is likely that the process of phagocytosis will be influenced by membrane structure, in particular by the fluidity of the membrane; the latter property can be influenced by the fatty acid composition of membrane phospholipids. Early studies indicated that phagocytosis by macrophages can be influenced by the fatty acid composition of the medium in which they are cultured [26, 28, 29]. Calder et al. [30] found that macrophages enriched with myristic or palmitic acids showed decreased rates of uptake of opsonised and unopsonised zymosan while those enriched with linoleic, α-linolenic, arachidonic, eicosapentaenoic or docosahexaenoic acids showed increased phagocytic activity. There was a strong positive correlation between phagocytosis and % PUFA, the ratio of unsaturated to saturated fatty acids and the index of unsaturation of the cellular phospholipids.

There are now several reports that dietary fish oil does not affect phagocytosis of cells or particles by monocytes or macrophages of various origins (see Tab. 6 for details). However, Eicher and McVey [58] found that fish oil feeding reduced the ability of murine Kupffer cells to phagocytose *Salmonella typhimurium*, although this was not associated with a reduced capacity of the cells to kill the bacteria. If the Kupffer cells were taken from mice infected with *Salmonella typhimurium* there was no apparent effect of previous diet on either phagocytosis or bacterial killing. These observations contrast with D'Ambola et al. [56] who showed that fish oil administered by gastric tube significantly diminishes the ability of neonatal rabbits to clear a challenge of *Staphylococcus aureus*.

Effects of *n*-3 PUFAs on expression of surface markers by mononuclear phagocytes

MHC expression

Macrophages present intracellular antigens to the T-cell receptor via the major histocompatibility class II antigen (MHC II); excess expression of MHC II may be involved in chronic inflammation and autoimmunity where there is an inappropriate response to host antigens. Incubation with DHA inhibits interleukin-4 (IL-4)- or IFN-γ-induced cell surface expression of MHC II (in the mouse these antigens are termed Ia) on mouse peritoneal macrophages [59]; DHA was more inhibitory than EPA and other 20-carbon fatty acids, and acted by inhibiting the increase in Ia mRNA which occurs after stimulation of macrophages with cytokines [59]. Recently, Hughes et al. [60] examined the effect of incubation of purified human monocytes with either EPA or DHA upon expression of MHC II, which is termed human leukocyte antigen (HLA): the proportion of monocytes expressing HLA-DP, -DQ or -DR was unaffected by incubation with EPA although there was a reduction in the level of expression of HLA-DR. EPA and DHA both reduced the proportion of HLA-DR or -DP positive monocytes following incubation with IFN-γ; the level of expression of these molecules on the monocyte surface was also reduced [60].

Inclusion of *n*-3 PUFAs in the diet of mice or rats results in a diminished percentage of peritoneal exudate cells bearing MHC II antigens on their surface [61–63]. Huang et al. [63] also reported that the level of MHC II expression on positive cells was suppressed by fish oil feeding. Feeding weanling rats a diet containing 200 g/kg fish oil for 12 weeks resulted in a decreased level of MHC II expression on thioglycollate-elicited peritoneal macrophages [64]. In accordance with these animal studies, Hughes et al. [65] reported that supplementation of the diet of human volunteers with *n*-3 PUFAs for 3 weeks resulted in a decreased level of MHC II (HLA-DP, -DQ and -DR) expression on the surface of peripheral blood monocytes.

Adhesion molecule expression

Adhesion molecules are involved in the movement of mononuclear phagocytes and other leukocytes between body compartments and into sites of immune or inflammatory activity. Excess expression of adhesion molecules on leukocytes and/or endothelial cells is associated with chronic inflammatory and autoimmune diseases. Calder et al. [30] reported that murine thioglycollate-elicited peritoneal macrophages cultured in the presence of EPA or DHA were less adherent to artificial surfaces (the adhesion to one of these surfaces is mediated by leukocyte function associated molecule-1 or LFA-1) than those cultured with some other fatty acids; α-linolenic acid was without effect. Recently, Hughes et al. [60] examined the effect of incubation of purified human monocytes with either EPA or DHA upon expression of intercellular adhesion molecule-1 (ICAM-1 or CD54). The proportion of monocytes expressing ICAM-1 was reduced by incubation with EPA and there was also a reduction in the level of expression of ICAM-1; DHA did not affect ICAM-1 or LFA-1 expression on resting monocytes. Both EPA and DHA reduced the proportion of ICAM-1 positive monocytes following incubation with IFN-γ; the level of expression of these molecules was also reduced [60]. DHA also reduced the expression of LFA-1 on IFN-γ-stimulated monocytes.

Feeding rats a fish oil-rich diet for 10 to 12 weeks resulted in a 30% reduction in the level of expression of CD18 (the β-chain of LFA-1) on thioglycollate-elicited peritoneal macrophages [64]. Supplementation of the human diet with *n*-3 PUFAs resulted in significantly lower levels of expression of ICAM-1 and LFA-1 on peripheral blood monocytes [65]. These observations suggest that fish oil feeding might affect the movement of macrophages and monocytes between body compartments and perhaps into sites of inflammatory or immune activity.

Effects of *n*-3 PUFAs on monocyte chemotaxis

Chemotaxis of blood monocytes towards the chemoattractants LTB_4 and fMLP was found to be suppressed following supplementation of the human diet with approximately 5.5 g EPA plus DHA for six weeks [40, 41, 66]. A recent study reported no effect of a lower dose of *n*-3 PUFAs (0.65 g/day for 12 weeks) upon monocyte chemotaxis towards pooled human serum [67].

Effects of *n*-3 PUFAs on cytokine production

Roles of macrophage-derived cytokines

Cytokines are soluble protein mediators produced by cells following their activation with specific stimuli. Cytokines act in an autocrine or paracrine manner to influence the activity of cell types which express specific receptors to which they can bind. Tumour necrosis factor (TNF)-α is the first cytokine released in response to bacterial endotoxin (or LPS). It is produced mainly by activated monocytes and macrophages. TNF activates neutrophils, monocytes and macrophages to initiate bacterial and tumour cell killing, increases adhesion molecule expression on the surface of neutrophils and endothelial cells, stimulates T- and B-cell function, up-regulates major histocompatibility antigens and initiates the production of other pro-inflammatory cytokines such as IL-1 and IL-6. Thus, TNF is a mediator of both natural and acquired immunity and an important link between specific immune responses and acute inflammation. In addition, TNF-α mediates the systemic effects of inflammation such as fever and hepatic acute phase protein synthesis. Production of small amounts of TNF is clearly beneficial in response to infection but overproduction can be dangerous and TNF is implicated in causing some of the pathological responses which occur in endotoxic shock, adult respiratory distress syndrome and other inflammatory conditions.

IL-1 appears to be the second cytokine released in response to inflammatory stimuli, including LPS and TNF, and it shares many of the pro-inflammatory effects of TNF (see [19]). Again, IL-1 is produced mainly by activated monocytes and macrophages. There are two IL-1 subtypes, α and β, which have similar biological activities and share cell surface receptors. IL-1 stimulates T and B lymphocyte proliferation and release of other cytokines (e.g. IL-2, IL-6) and induces hypotension, fever, weight loss, neutrophilia and the acute phase response.

IL-6 is produced by activated monocytes and macrophages in response to IL-1 and TNF. It has a wide range of activities, many of them shared with TNF and IL-1 (see [19]). IL-6 modulates T- and B-cell function and is found in the bloodstream of patients with sepsis, burns and trauma.

Animal studies

A number of animal studies have investigated the effect of dietary lipids upon *ex vivo* production of macrophage-derived cytokines, including TNF, IL-1 and IL-6. These studies have been reviewed in detail elsewhere [19]. These studies differ greatly in the protocols used; they have varied in the amount of fat given (50 to 200 g/kg) and the duration of feeding (2 to 15 weeks), the nature of the dietary comparisons being made (to chow, to other high fat diets), the species of animal used (mouse, rat, pig), the type of macrophage used (alveolar, peritoneal, Kupffer, peripheral blood) and its state of activation at harvesting (monocyte, resident macrophage, elicited macrophage), the agent used to elicit macrophages (thioglycollate, casein, complete Freund's adjuvant (CFA)), the stimulus used to induce cytokine production (LPS, another cytokine) and its concentration, the type of serum present in *ex vivo* macrophage culture (none, fetal calf, autologous) and its concentration, and the duration of *ex vivo* macrophage culture (see [19] for details). Other technical differences between studies have been discussed elsewhere [19].

Several studies have reported that feeding rodents *n*-3 PUFA-containing oils results in enhanced production of TNF by macrophages *ex vivo*, although there are reports of decreased production or no effect following fish or linseed oil feeding. These differences between studies appear not to relate to species, duration of feeding or type or amount of *n*-3 PUFA in the diet. However, there may be some relationship with the state of activation of the macrophages used. All studies which have used murine resident peritoneal macrophages, one study using rat resident alveolar

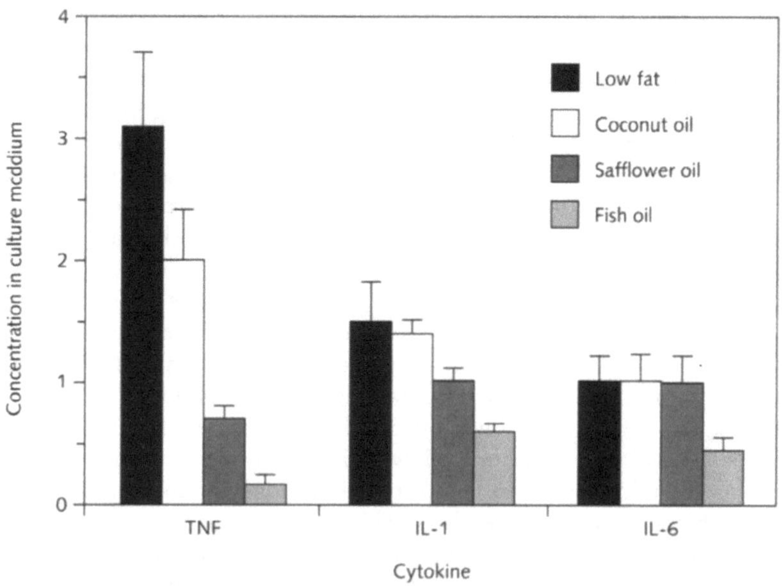

Figure 2
Effect of dietary lipids on the production of cytokines by murine peritoneal macrophages. Mice were fed on a low fat (25 g/kg corn oil) diet or on diets containing 200 g/kg of either hydrogenated coconut oil, safflower oil or fish oil. Thioglycollate-elicited peritoneal macrophages were prepared and cultured with bacterial LPS (10 μg/ml) for 24 hours. The medium was collected and cytokine concentrations were measured by ELISA; concentrations are expressed as ng/ml (TNF-α), ng/10 ml (IL-1β) or ng/0.1 ml (IL-6). TNF-α and IL-1β data are from [74] and IL-6 data are from [43].

macrophages and one study using rat resident peritoneal macrophages report an enhancing effect of *n*-3 PUFAs upon TNF production [32, 35, 45, 55, 68, 71]; only one study which used rat resident peritoneal macrophages has reported reduced TNF production following fish oil feeding [49]. Three studies report that *n*-3 PUFA-rich diets do not affect TNF production by CFA-elicited peritoneal macrophages from rats or mice [32, 35, 70]. The effect of dietary *n*-3 PUFAs upon TNF production by thioglycollate-elicited peritoneal macrophages is unclear with studies reporting no effect [35, 54, 72, 73], reduction [43, 52, 74] (Fig. 2) or enhancement [54, 72]. Comparison of the outcome of these studies is complicated by the different procedures used for *ex vivo* culture of the cells (see [19] for discussion). The only animal study which has investigated TNF production by peripheral blood mononuclear cells (PBMCs) showed decreased production following the infusion of a 10% (v/v) fish oil emulsion [75]; this is an interesting observation since it agrees with the findings of a number of studies using human PBMCs (see below). In addition to studies measuring TNF production *ex vivo*, it was reported that feeding mice *n*-3 PUFA-rich diets resulted in reduced ability of elicited peritoneal macrophages to kill L929 cells [44, 52]; L929 cells are killed by TNF and so the reduced cytotoxicity of macrophages towards these cells suggests a reduced ability to produce TNF.

Some studies have investigated the effects of dietary lipids upon circulating TNF levels which would reflect *in vivo* production of the cytokine. Watanabe et al. [35] found that TNF levels were significantly higher in the plasma of LPS-injected (10 mg/kg body weight) mice fed diets containing 100 g/kg perilla oil than in the plasma of those fed 100 g/kg safflower oil. Similarly, Chang et al. [71] reported higher serum TNF levels 1 and 1.5 hours following intraperitoneal injection of LPS (10 μg) into fish oil fed-mice compared with those fed coconut or corn oil. Blok et al. [69] also found higher circulating levels of TNF after intraperitoneal injection of LPS (10 μg) in fish oil-fed mice compared with those fed laboratory chow or a diet rich in corn oil. These observations are not incompatible with the *ex vivo* observations since in these studies LPS was injected into animals which had received no previous challenge; thus among mononuclear phagocytes, the likely responding cells would be resident macrophages which appear to produce increased levels of TNF following fish oil feeding (see above). A different situation might be encountered if LPS or another immunological challenge was provided to animals whose macrophages had already been activated in some way. This might be important in the context of chronic inflammatory or autoimmune disease where activated macrophages exist in the circulation and at sites of immune reactivity.

All studies which have used thioglycollate-elicited peritoneal macrophages and the only study to use Kupffer cells report that dietary fish oil results in decreased *ex vivo* production of IL-1 [43, 73, 74, 76] (Fig. 2). In contrast, two studies have reported that fish oil enhances IL-1 production by murine resident macrophages [68, 69]. In addition, Ertel et al. [77] showed that the reduction in *ex vivo* IL-1 production by resident peritoneal macrophages which accompanies haemorragic shock in corn or safflower oil-fed mice was prevented by fish oil feeding. This study also showed no difference in IL-1 production by resident peritoneal macrophages taken from sham-operated mice fed these three diets [77].

There are no studies reporting the effect of dietary fatty acids upon IL-6 production by resident peritoneal macrophages. One study using murine thioglycollate-elicited peritoneal macrophages showed a significant reduction in LPS-stimulated IL-6 production following fish oil feeding [43] (Fig. 2); production following stimulation of the cells with TNF was also significantly reduced (P. Yaqoob and P.C. Calder, unpublished observations). Rat PBMCs showed reduced IL-6 production following fish oil infusion for 4 days [75]. These studies are supported by the *in vitro* observation that EPA and DHA inhibit IL-6 production by rat thioglycollate-elicited peritoneal macrophages [78].

Despite the apparent contradictions in the literature regarding the effects of feeding animals *n*-3 PUFA-rich diets upon proinflammatory cytokine production some patterns do emerge. It appears that fish oil feeding enhances TNF and IL-1 production by resident macrophages. In contrast, fish oil feeding appears to reduce TNF, IL-1 and IL-6 production by thioglycollate-elicited macrophages and by PBMCs. Possible reasons for different responses of these cell types to dietary *n*-3 PUFAs have been presented elsewhere [19].

Human studies

A large number of studies have investigated the effect of supplementation of the diet of healthy subjects with *n*-3 PUFAs, upon *ex vivo* PBMC cytokine production (see Tab. 7): studies have also been performed in patients with rheumatoid arthritis, inflammatory skin diseases, type-1 diabetes and multiple sclerosis (Tab. 7). A number of studies have shown that supplementation of the diet of healthy humans with between 1.1 and 5 g EPA + DHA per day for a number of weeks leads to a significant reduction in *ex vivo* production of TNF [41, 80, 83, 84, 86], IL-1 [41, 80–84, 86] and IL-6 [80, 82, 83] by PBMCs (see Tab. 7 for details). Recently it was reported that supplementation of the diet of healthy subjects with 0.5 g *n*-3 PUFAs per day for 12 weeks did not affect *ex vivo* production of TNF-α, IL-1β or IL-6 by PBMCs [67].

The effects of dietary α-linolenic acid upon IL-1β and TNFα production by human cells have been reported; subjects consumed a sunflower oil-rich diet (which was very similar to their typical diet) or a diet rich in α-linolenic acid which was provided by linseed oil capsules and linseed oil-based spreads and cooking oils [86]. In this way the linseed oil consumption increased to a mean of 13.7 g/day. *Ex vivo* production of both IL-1β and TNFα by PBMCs was decreased by the linseed oil diet [86]. If the subjects then supplemented their diet with encapsulated EPA plus DHA production of both cytokines was further decreased [86]. These authors showed a correlation between mononuclear cell EPA content and production of IL-1β and TNFα [86].

Supplementation of the diet of multiple sclerosis patients with encapsulated fish oil providing approximately 5 g EPA plus DHA per day for 24 weeks resulted in lower *ex vivo* production of IL-1β and TNFα by PBMCs [84]. An earlier study reported lower production of IL-1 by PBMCs taken from rheumatoid arthritis patients who had consumed *n*-3 PUFAs for 24 weeks [79].

Table 7 - Summary of studies investigating the effects of n-3 *PUFAs on* ex vivo *pro-inflammatory cytokine production by human mononuclear cells.*

Subjects	Details of supplementation used	Stimulus	Cytokine	Observations	Ref.
Healthy men	Encapsulated *n*-3 PUFAs (2.75 g EPA + 1.85 g DHA per day); 6 weeks	LPS	IL-1α	Decreased production (not significant); decreased production 10 weeks post-supplementation; production returned to normal 20 weeks post-supplementation	41
			IL-1β	Decreased production at end of supplementation and 10 weeks post-supplementation; production returned to normal 20 weeks post-supplementation	
			TNF	Decreased production (not significant); decreased production 10 weeks post-supplementation; production returned to normal 20 weeks post-supplementation	
Rheumatoid arthritis patients; men and women	Encapsulated olive oil (9 g/day) or fish oil (27 mg/kg body weight EPA + 18 mg/kg body weight DHA per day or 54 mg/kg body weight EPA + 36 mg/kg body weight DHA per day); 24 weeks	LPS	IL-1	Decreased production in all groups; decrease greater in "high" *n*-3 PUFA group	79
Healthy women	Encapsulated *n*-3 PUFAs (1.68 g EPA + 0.72 g DHA per day); 4, 8 or 12 weeks	LPS	IL-1β	Time-dependent decrease in production in older women; non-significant decrease in production in younger women	80
			TNF	Time dependent decrease in production in both young and old women.	
		Con A	IL-6	Time dependent decrease in production in both young and old women; decrease greater in older women	

Table 7 (continued)

Subjects	Details of supplementation used	Stimulus	Cytokine	Observations	Ref.
Healthy or type-1 diabetic men	Encapsulated *n*-3 PUFAs (2.04 g EPA + 1.14 g DHA or 1.02 g EPA + 0.57 g DHA per day) or placebo (6 or 3 g oil mix/day); 7 weeks	LPS	TNFα	No effect	81
			IL-1β	No effect on secreted IL-1β	
				No effect of lower *n*-3 PUFA dose on on intracellular IL-1β	
				Higher *n*-3 PUFA dose decreased intracellular levels of IL-1β in response to all concentrations of LPS in both mononuclear cell and monocyte cultures; no difference between subject groups	
Healthy men and women	Encapsulated *n*-3 PUFAs (0.7 to 0.94 g EPA + 0.46 to 0.62 g DHA per day); 6–8 weeks	LPS	IL-1	Decreased production in response to low concentrations (≤ 0.001 μg/ml) of LPS	82
			IL-6	Decreased production in response to low concentrations (≤ 0.001 μg/ml) of LPS	
			TNFα	No effect	
Healthy men	Low fat, low cholesterol diet or low fat, low cholesterol diet + fish-rich diet (1.23 g *n*-3 PUFA/day); 24 weeks	LPS	IL-1β	Decreased production in the fish group	83
			TNF	Decreased production in the fish group	
		Con A	IL-6	Decreased production in the fish group	
Healthy or multiple sclerosis patients; men and women	Encapsulated *n*-3 PUFAs (3.1 g EPA + 1.86 g DHA per day); 4 to 24 weeks	LPS	IL-1β	Decreased production at 4, 12 and 24 weeks; return to baseline production by 12 weeks post-supplementation; no difference between subject groups	84
			TNFα	Decreased production at 4, 12 and 24 weeks; return to baseline production by 12 weeks post-supplementation; no difference between subject groups	

Table 7 (continued)

Subjects	Details of supplementation used	Stimulus	Cytokine	Observations	Ref.
Psoriasis or atopic dermatitis patients; genders not given	Encapsulated *n*-3 PUFA ethyl esters (3.06 g EPA + 1.92 g DHA per day) or encapsulated corn oil (6 g/day); 16 weeks	PHA	IL-6	No effect	85
			TNF	Increased production with corn oil	
Healthy men and women	Encapsulated fish oil (0.5 g EPA + DHA per day); 12 weeks	LPS	TNFα	No effect	67
			IL-1β	No effect	
			IL-6	No effect	
Healthy men	Sunflower oil-rich diet or linseed oil-rich diet (mean of 13.7 g α-linolenic acid per day) [α-linolenic acid provided as linseed oil capsules and linseed oil-based spreads and cooking oil]; 4 weeks	LPS	TNFα	No effect of sunflower oil; decreased production with linseed oil	86
			IL-1β	No effect of sunflower oil; decreased production with linseed oil	
	Sunflower oil-rich diet or linseed oil-rich diet (mean of 13.7 g α-linolenic acid per day) plus encapsulated *n*-3 PUFAs (1.62 g EPA + 1.08 g DHA per day); 4 weeks	LPS	TNFα	Decreased production	
			IL-1β	Decreased production	

Con A indicates concanavalin A; PHA indicates phytohaemagglutinin

Conclusion

The production of macrophage-derived proinflammatory eicosanoids such as PGE_2 is markedly reduced by feeding diets rich in *n*-3 PUFAs. Furthermore, inclusion in the diet of high levels of *n*-3 PUFAs significantly reduces the movement of human monocytes towards chemotactic agents and the production of proinflammatory cytokines by human mononuclear phagocytes. There are a number of contradictory observations regarding the effects of dietary *n*-3 PUFAs on production of proinflammatory cytokines by animal macrophages; these most likely relate to the different experimental protocols used. *n*-3 PUFAs also appear to reduce adhesion molecule expression and thus might influence the movement of mononuclear phagocytes between body compartments. Several studies indicate a reduction of MHC II expression on mononuclear phagocytes following fish oil feeding; this would suggest a dimished ability to present antigen. There is no clear consensus regarding the effects of *n*-3 PUFA consumption on the generation of reactive oxygen and nitrogen species and on macrophage-mediated phagocytosis. Although some of the effects of *n*-3 PUFAs may be brought about by modulation of the amount and types of eicosanoids made, it is likely that these fatty acids can also elicit their effects by eicosanoid-independent mechanisms. Such *n*-3 PUFA-induced effects may be of use as a therapy for acute and chronic inflammation and for disorders which involve an inappropriately-activated immune response.

References

1 Auger MJ, Ross JA (1992) The biology of the macrophage. In: CE Lewis, J O'D McGee (eds): *The macrophage*. IRL Press, Oxford, 1–74
2 Gendelman HE, Morahan PS (1992) Macrophages in viral infections. In: CE Lewis, J O'D McGee (eds): *The macrophage*. IRL Press, Oxford, 157–213
3 Speert DP (1992) Macrophages in bacterial infection. In: CE Lewis, J O'D McGee (eds): *The macrophage*. IRL Press, Oxford, 215–263
4 Sadick MD (1992) Macrophages in parasitic infection. In: CE Lewis, J O'D McGee (eds): *The macrophage*. IRL Press, Oxford, 265–284
5 Rees RC, Parry H (1992) Macrophages in tumour immunity. In: CE Lewis, J O'D McGee (eds): *The macrophage*. IRL Press, Oxford, 315–357
6 Pollack S, Etzioni A (1992) Macrophages in autoimmunity and primary immunodeficiency. In: CE Lewis, J O'D McGee (eds): *The macrophage*. IRL Press, Oxford, 285–313
7 Meade CJ, Mertin J (1978) Fatty acids and immunity. *Adv Lipid Res* 16: 127–165
8 Goldyne ME, Stobo JD (1981) Immunoregulatory role of prostaglandins and related lipids. *Crit Rev Immunol* 2: 189–223
9 Goodwin JS, Cueppens J (1983) Regulation of the immune response by prostaglandins. *J Clin Immunol* 3: 295–315

10 Roper RL, Phipps RP (1994) Prostaglandin E_2 regulation of the immune response. *Adv Prost Thromb Leuk Res* 22: 101–111
11 Hwang D (1989) Essential fatty acids and the immune response. *FASEB J* 3: 2052–2061
12 Kinsella JE, Lokesh B, Broughton S, Whelan J (1990) Dietary polyunsaturated fatty acids and eicosanoids: potential effects on the modulation of inflammatory and immune cells: An overview. *Nutrition* 6: 24–44
13 Calder PC (1996) Effects of fatty acids and dietary lipids on cells of the immune system. *Proc Nutr Soc* 55: 127–150
14 Calder PC (1996) Can *n*-3 polyunsaturated fatty acids be used as immunomodulatory agents? *Biochem Soc Trans* 24: 211–220
15 Calder PC (1996) Immunomodulatory and anti-inflammatory effects of *n*-3 polyunsaturated fatty acids. *Proc Nutr Soc* 55: 737–774
16 Gurr MI (1983) The role of lipids in the regulation of the immune system. *Prog Lipid Res* 22: 257–287
17 Peck MD (1994) Interactions of lipids with immune function II: Experimental and clinical studies of lipids and immunity. *J Nutr Biochem* 5: 514–521
18 Calder PC (1995) Fatty acids, dietary lipids and lymphocyte functions. *Biochem Soc Trans* 23: 302–309
19 Calder PC (1997) N-3 polyunsaturated fatty acids and cytokine production in health and disease. *Ann Nutr Metab* 41: 203–234
20 Calder PC (1998) Dietary fatty acids and the immune system. *Nutr Rev* 56: 570–583
21 Miles EA, Calder PC (1998) Modulation of immune function by dietary fatty acids. *Proc Nutr Soc* 57: 277–292
22 Blok WL, Katan MB, van der Meer JWM (1996) Modulation of inflammation and cytokine production by dietary (*n*-3) fatty acids. *J Nutr* 126: 1515–1533
23 Calder PC (1998) Dietary fatty acids and lymphocyte functions. *Proc Nutr Soc; in press*
24 Meydani SN (1996) Effect of (*n*-3) polyunsaturated fatty acids on cytokine production and their biologic function. *Nutrition* 12: S8–S14
25 Endres S, von Schacky C (1996) *n*-3 Polyunsaturated fatty acids and human cytokine synthesis. *Curr Opin Lipidol* 7: 48–52
26 Lokesh BR, Wrann M (1984) Incorporation of palmitic acid or oleic acid into macrophage membrane lipids exerts differential effects on the function of normal mouse peritoneal macrophages. *Biochim Biophys Acta* 792: 141-148
27 Lokesh BR, Black JM, German JB, Kinsella JE (1988) Docosahexaenoic acid and other dietary omega-3 polyunsaturated fatty acids suppress leukotriene synthesis by mouse peritoneal macrophages. *Lipids* 23: 968–972
28 Schroit AJ, Gallily R (1979) Macrophage fatty acid composition and phagocytosis: Effect of unsaturation on cellular phagocytic activity. *Immunology* 36: 199–205
29 Mahoney EM, Hamill AL, Scott WA, Cohn ZA (1977) Response of endocytosis to altered fatty acyl composition of macrophage phospholipids. *Proc Natl Acad Sci USA* 74: 4895–4899
30 Calder PC, Bond JA, Harvey DJ,.Gordon S, Newsholme EA (1990) Uptake of saturat-

ed and unsaturated fatty acids into macrophage lipids and their effect upon macrophage adhesion and phagocytosis. *Biochem J* 269: 807–814

31 Magrum LJ, Johnston PV (1983) Modulation of prostaglandin synthesis in rat peritoneal macrophages with ω-3 fatty acids. *Lipids* 18: 514–521

32 Hardardottir I, Kinsella JE (1992) Increasing the dietary (*n*-3) to (*n*-6) polyunsaturated fatty acid ratio increases tumor necrosis factor production by murine resident peritoneal macrophages without an effect on elicited peritoneal macrophages. *J Nutr* 122: 1942–1951

33 Lokesh BR, Hsieh HL, Kinsella JE (1986) Peritoneal macrophages from mice fed dietary (*n*-3) polyunsaturated fatty acids secrete low levels of prostaglandins. *J Nutr* 116: 2547–2552

34 Chapkin RS, Akoh CC, Lewis RE (1992) Dietary fish oil modulation of *in vivo* peritoneal macrophage leukotriene production and phagocytosis. *J Nutr Biochem* 3: 599–604

35 Watanabe S, Hayashi H, Onozaki K, Okuyama H (1991) Effect of dietary α-linolenate/linoleate balance on lipopolysaccharide-induced tumor necrosis factor production in mouse macrophages. *Life Sci* 48: 2013–2020

36 Brouard C, Pascaud M (1990) Effects of moderate dietary supplementations with *n*-3 fatty acids on macrophage and lymphocyte phospholipids and macrophage eicosanoid synthesis in the rat. *Biochim Biophys Acta* 1047: 19–28

37 Sherrington EJ, Harvey DJ, Calder PC (1995) The effect of dietary lipid manipulation on macrophage phospholipid fatty acid composition and membrane fluidity. *Proc Nutr Soc* 54: 121A

38 Surette ME, Whelan J, Lu G, Hardardottir I, Kinsella JE (1995) Dietary *n*-3 polyunsaturated fatty acids modify Syrian hampster platelet and macrophage phospholipid fatty acyl composition and eicosanoid synthesis: a controlled study. *Biochim Biophys Acta* 122: 185–191

39 Fritsche KL, Alexander DW, Cassity NA, Huang S-C (1993) Maternally supplied fish oil alters piglet immune cell fatty acid profile and eicosanoid production. *Lipids* 28: 677–682

40 Lee TH, Hoover RL, Williams JD, Sperling RI, Ravalese J, Spur BW, Robinson DR, Corey EJ, Lewis RA, Austen KF (1985) Effects of dietary enrichment with EPA and DHA on *in vitro* neutrophil and monocyte leukotriene generation and neutrophil function. *New Engl J Med* 312: 1217–1224

41 Endres S, Ghorbani R, Kelley VE, Georgilis K, Lonnemann G, van der Meer JMW, Cannon, JG, Rogers TS, Klempner MS, Weber PC, Schaeffer EJ, Wolff SM, Dinarello CA (1989) The effect of dietary supplementation with *n*-3 polyunsaturated fatty acids on the synthesis of interleukin-1 and tumor necrosis factor by mononuclear cells. *New Eng J Med* 320: 265–271

42 Halvorsen DA, Hansen J-B, Grimsgaard S, Bonaa KH, Kierulf P, Nordoy A (1997) The effect of highly purified eicosapentaenoic and docosahexaenoic acids on monocyte phagocytosis in man. *Lipids* 32: 935–942

43 Yaqoob P, Calder PC (1995) Effects of dietary lipid manipulation upon inflammatory mediator production by murine macrophages. *Cell Immunol* 163: 120–128
44 Black JM, Kinsella JE (1993) Dietary *n*-3 fatty acids alter mouse peritoneal macrophage cytotoxicity. *Ann Nutr Metab* 37: 110–120
45 Hardardottir I, Kinsella JE (1991) Tumour necrosis factor production by murine resident peritoneal macrophages is enhanced by dietary *n*-3 polyunsaturated fatty acids. *Biochim Biophys Acta* 1095: 187–195
46 Chapkin RS, Hubbard NE, Erickson KL (1990) 5-Series peptido-leukotriene synthesis in mouse peritoneal macrophages: modulation by dietary *n*-3 fatty acids. *Biochem Biophys Res Commun* 171: 764–769
47 Fisher M, Levine PH, Weiner BH, Johnson MH, Doyle EM, Ellis PA, Hoogasian JJ (1990) Dietary *n*-3 fatty acid supplementation reduces superoxide production and chemiluminescence in a monocyte-enriched preparation of leukocytes. *Am J Clin Nutr* 51: 804–808
48 Joe B, Lokesh BR (1994) Role of capsaicin, curcumin and dietary *n*-3 fatty acids in lowering the generation of reactive oxygen species in rat peritoneal macrophages. *Biochim Biophys Acta* 1224: 255–263
49 Boutard V, Fouquery B, Philippe C, Perez J, Baud L (1994) Fish oil supplementation and essential fatty acid deficiency reduce nitric oxide synthesis by rat macrophages. *Kidney Int* 46: 1280–1286
50 Babu US, Bunning VK, Wiesenfeld P, Raybourne RB, O'Donnell M (1997) Effect of dietary flaxseed on fatty acid composition, superoxide, nitric oxide generation and antilisterial activity of peritoneal macrophages from female Sprague-Dawley rats. *Life Sci* 60: 545–554
51 Hubbard NE, Somers SD, Erickson KL (1991) Effect of dietary fish oil on development and selected functions of murine inflammatory macrophages. *J Leuk Biol* 49: 592–598
52 Renier G, Skamene E, de Sanctis J, Radzioch D (1993) Dietary *n*-3 polyunsaturated fatty acids prevent the development of atherosclerotic lesions in mice: Modulation of macrophage secretory activities. *Arterio Thomb* 13: 1515–1524
53 Berger A, German JB, Chiang BL, Ansari AA, Keen CL, Fletcher MP, Gershwin MR (1993) Influence of feeding unsaturated fats on growth and immune status of mice. *J Nutr* 123: 225–233
54 Hubbard NE, Chapkin RS, Erickson KL (1994) Effect of dietary linseed oil on tumoricidal activity and eicosanoid production in murine macrophages. *Lipids* 29: 651–655
55 Chaet MS, Garcia VF, Arya G, Ziegler MM (1994) Dietary fish oil enhances macrophage production of nitric oxide. *J Surg Res* 57: 65–68
56 D'Ambola JB, Aeberhard EE, Trang N, Gaffar S, Barrett CT, Sherman MP (1991) Effect of dietary (*n*–3) and (*n*-6) fatty acids on *in vivo* pulmonary bacterial clearance by neonatal rabbits. *J Nutr* 121: 1262–1269
57 Turek JJ, Schoenlein IA, Clark LK, van Alstine WG (1994) Dietary polyunsaturated fatty acids effects on immune cells of the porcine lung. *J Leuk Biol* 56: 599–604

58 Eicher SD, McVey DS (1995) Dietary modulation of Kupffer cell and splenocyte function during a *Salmonella typhimurium* challenge in mice. *J Leuk Biol* 58: 32–39

59 Khair-El-Din TA, Sicher SC, Vazquez MA, Wright WJ, Lu CY (1995) Docosahexaenoic acid, a major constituent of fetal serum and fish oil diets, inhibits IFNγ-induced Ia-expression by murine macrophages *in vitro*. *J Immunol* 154: 1296–1306

60 Hughes DA, Southon S, Pinder AC (1996) (*n*-3) Polyunsaturated fatty acids modulate the expression of functionally associated molecules on human monocytes *in vitro*. *J Nutr* 126: 603–610

61 Kelley VE, Ferretti A, Izui S, Strom TB (1985) A fish oil diet rich in eicosapentaenoic acid reduces cyclooxygenase metabolites and suppresses lupus in MRL-lpr mice. *J Immunol* 134: 1914–1919

62 Mosquera J, Rodriguez-Iturbe B, Parra G (1990) Fish oil dietary supplementation reduces Ia expression in rat and mouse peritoneal macrophages. *Clin Immunol Immunopathol* 56: 124–129

63 Huang S-C, Misfeldt ML, Fritsche KL (1992) Dietary fat influences Ia antigen expression and immune cell populations in the murine peritoneum and spleen. *J Nutr* 122: 1219–1231

64 Sherrington EJ, Sanderson P, Calder PC (1995) The effect of dietary lipid manipulation on macrophage cell surface molecule expression. *Biochem Soc Trans* 23: 272S

65 Hughes DA, Pinder AC, Piper Z, Johnson IT, Lund EK (1996) Fish oil supplementation inhibits the expression of major histocompatibility complex class II molecules and adhesion molecules on human monocytes. *Am J Clin Nutr* 63: 267–272

66 Schmidt EB, Varming K, Pederson JO, Lervang HH, Grunnet N, Jersild C, Dyerberg J (1992) Long term supplementation with *n*-3 fatty acids. II. Effect on neutrophil and monocyte chemotaxis. *Scand J Clin Lab Invest* 52: 229–236

67 Schmidt EB, Varming K, Moller JM, Bulow Pederson I, Madsen P, Dyerberg J (1996) No effect of a very low dose of *n*-3 fatty acids on monocyte function in healthy humans. *Scand J Clin Invest* 56: 87–92

68 Lokesh BR, Sayers TJ, Kinsella JE (1990) Interleukin-1 and tumor necrosis factor synthesis by mouse peritoneal macrophages is enhanced by dietary *n*-3 polyunsaturated fatty acids. *Immunol Lett* 23: 281–286

69 Blok WL, de Bruijn MFTR, Leenan PJM, Elinh WMC, van Rooijen N, Stanley ER, Buurman WA, van der Meer JWM (1996) Dietary *n*-3 fatty acids increase spleen size and postendotoxin circulating TNF in mice; Role of macrophages, macrophage precursors, and colony-stimulating-factor-1. *J Immunol* 157: 5569–5573

70 Turek JJ, Schoenlein IA, Bottoms GD (1991) The effect of dietary *n*-3 and *n*-6 fatty acids on tumor necrosis factor-α production and leucine aminopeptidase levels in rat peritoneal macrophages. *Prost Leuk Ess Fatty Acids* 43: 141–149

71 Chang HR, Arsenijevic D, Pechere JC, Piguet PF, Mensi N, Girardier L, Dulloo AG (1992) Dietary supplementation with fish oil enhances *in vivo* synthesis of tumor necrosis factor. *Immunol Lett* 34: 13–18

72 Somers SD, Erickson KL (1994) Alteration of tumor necrosis factor-α production by

macrophages from mice fed diets high in eicosapentaenoic and docosahexaenoic acids. *Cell Immunol* 153: 287–297

73 Tappia PS, Grimble RF (1994) Complex modulation of cytokine induction by endotoxin and tumour necrosis factor from peritoneal macrophages of rats by diets containing fats of different saturated, monounsaturated and polyunsaturated fatty acid composition. *Clin Sci* 87: 173–178

74 Wallace FA, Neeley SJ, Miles EA, Calder PC (1997) Dietary fish oil decreases the production of pro-inflammatory mediators by murine macrophages. *Proc Nutr Soc* 57: 50A

75 Grimm H, Tibell A, Norrlind B, Blecher C, Wilker S, Schwemmle K (1994) Immunoregulation by parenteral lipids: impact of the *n*-3 to *n*-6 fatty acid ratio. *J Parent Ent Nutr* 18: 417–421

76 Billiar T, Bankey P, Svingen B, Curran RD, West MA, Holman RT, Simmons RL, Cerra, FB (1988) Fatty acid uptake and Kupffer cell function: fish oil alters eicosanoid and monokine production to endotoxin stimulation. *Surgery* 104: 343–349

77 Ertel W, Morrison MH, Ayala A, Chaudry IH (1993) Modulation of macrophage membrane phospholipids by *n*-3 polyunsaturated fatty acids increases interleukin 1 release and prevents suppression of cellular immunity following hemorrhagic shock. *Arch Surg* 128: 15–21

78 Tappia PS, Man WJ, Grimble RF (1995) Influence of unsaturated fatty acids on the production of tumour necrosis factor and interleukin-6 by rat peritoneal macrophages. *Mol Cell Biochem* 143: 89–98

79 Kremer JM, Lawrence DA, Jubiz W, Di Giacomo R, Rynes K, Bartholomew LE, Sherman M (1990) Dietary fish oil and olive oil supplementation in patients with rheumatoid arthritis. *Arth Rheum* 33: 810–820

80 Meydani SN, Endres S, Woods MM, Goldin BR, Soo C, Morrill-Labrode A, Dinarello C, Gorbach SL (1991) Oral (*n*-3) fatty acid supplementation suppresses cytokine production and lymphocyte proliferation: comparison between young and older women. *J Nutr* 121: 547–555

81 Molvig J, Pociot F, Worsaae H, Wogensen LD, Baek L, Christensen P, Mandrup-Poulsen T, Andersen K, Madsen P, Dyerberg J, Nerup J (1991) Dietary supplementation with ω-3 polyunsaturated fatty acids decreases mononuclear cell proliferation and interleukin-1β content but not monokine secretion in healthy and insulin-dependent diabetic individuals. Scand J Immunol 34: 399–410

82 Cooper AL, Gibbons L, Horan MA, Little RA, Rothwell NJ (1993) Effect of dietary fish oil supplementation on fever and cytokine production in human volunteers. *Clin Nutr* 12: 321–328

83 Meydani SN, Lichtenstein AH, Cornwall S, Meydani M, Goldin BR, Rasmussen H, Dinarello CA, Schaefer EJ (1993) Immunologic effects of national cholesterol education panel step-2 diets with and without fish-derived *n*-3 fatty acid enrichement. *J Clin Invest* 92: 105–113

84 Gallai V, Sarchielli P, Trequattrini A, Franceschini M, Floridi A, Firenze C, Alberti A, Di Benedetto D, Stragliotto E (1993) Cytokine secretion and eicosanoid production in the

peripheral blood mononuclear cells of MS patients undergoing dietary supplementation with *n*-3 polyunsaturated fatty acids. *J Neuroimmunol* 56: 143–153

85 Soyland E, Lea T, Sandstad B, Drevon A (1994) Dietary supplementation with very long chain *n*-3 fatty acids in man decreases expression of the interleukin-2 receptor (CD25) on mitogen-stimulated lymphocytes from patients with inflammatory skin diseases. *Eur J Clin Invest* 24: 236–242

86 Caughey GE, Mantzioris E, Gibson RA, Cleland LG, James MJ (1996) The effect on human tumor necrosis factor α and interleukin 1β production of diets enriched in *n*-3 fatty acids from vegetable oil or fish oil. *Am J Clin Nutr* 63: 116–122

Gammalinolenic acid treatment of rheumatoid arthritis

Robert B. Zurier

University of Massachusetts Medical Center, 55 Lake Avenue North, Worcester,
MA 01655, USA

Introduction

Rheumatoid arthritis (RA) is a chronic systemic inflammatory disorder of unknown etiology affecting approximately 1% of the world's population [1]. It is a uniquely human disease characterized by symmetrical polyarthritis. Women are affected 2–3 times more often than men but this female preponderance is less impressive when one considers only those patients who are serologically positive for rheumatoid factor and are found to have radiographic evidence of erosive changes in joints [2]. RA can occur at any age; however, the incidence does increase with advancing age. RA seems to have no geographical limits; it occurs in every part of the world and its prevalence is not influenced by climate or temperature. The incidence in different studies varies from 4.2 to 26 per 10,000. Occasionally, several members of a family are found to have RA, and a greater than expected incidence occurs in monozygotic twins [3]. Genetic studies indicate an association of vulnerability to RA and severity of disease with the presence of a conserved sequence of amino acids in the third hypervariable region of the β1 chain of certain human leukocyte antigen (HLA) Class II molecules, HLA-DR4 and DR1 [4]. As Class II molecules are involved in antigen presentation, it is possible that further analysis will lead to identification of an infectious or chemical antigen that may be responsible for the initiation of RA.

Management of patients with RA has improved mainly through development of antiinflammatory drugs, advances in surgical repair and replacement of damaged joints, and more intelligent use of corticosteroids and other drugs such as methotrexate. Unfortunately, many of these interventions are associated with adverse effects that can be as difficult to manage as the disease itself. In addition, life expectancy is reduced to that of grade IV Hodgkins disease or untreated triple-vessel coronary artery disease in RA patients with severe disease [5]. Clearly, new ways to treat RA patients are needed.

Medicinal Fatty Acids in Inflammation, edited by J. Kremer

Fatty acid metabolism

Two families of fatty acids essential to the body must be obtained by dietary means. They include the *n*-6 series derived from linoleic acid (LA; 18:2*n*-6) and the *n*-3 series derived from α-linolenic acid (18:3*n*-3). Using this notation, 18 refers to the number of carbon atoms in the fatty acid; the degree of saturation (the number of double carbon-carbon bonds) follows the number of carbon atoms. The *n* refers to the number of carbon atoms from the methyl (omega) end of the fatty acid chain to the first double bond. The metabolic pathways of the *n*-6 fatty acids are shown in Figure 1. Examination of the pathway suggests that synthesis of gammalinolenic acid (GLA) from LA should be abundant. However, that does not seem to be the case, and the activity of Δ6 desaturase which converts LA to GLA is impaired in many disease states [6]. Therefore, if cellular proportions of GLA and subsequently dihomogammalinolenic acid (DGLA) are to be increased, GLA must be supplied exogenously. It also appears that increases in GLA should lead to increased synthesis of arachidonic acid (AA). Most studies [7], but not all [8], indicate that AA is not increased by GLA administration, probably because Δ5 desaturase activity, which converts DGLA to AA, is quite sluggish in humans.

The relationship between essential fatty acids and prostaglandins was discovered simultaneously and independently by van Dorp et al. [9] and Bergstrom et al. [10]. Both groups reported that AA was converted to prostaglandin E_2 (PGE_2) and shortly thereafter they showed that PGE_1 is formed from DGLA [11]. PGE_1 suppresses diverse effector systems of inflammation and reduces acute and chronic inflammation in several animal models [12]. In addition, PGE_1 suppresses synovial cell growth [13]. Also, non-steroidal anti-inflammatory drug (NSAID) induced down-regulation of the glucocorticoid receptor in human synovial fibroblasts, which limits the ability of corticosteroids to suppress metalloproteinase production, is prevented by a PGE_1 analog [14]. Moreover, intravenous PGE_1 suppresses human neutrophil activation [15] and reduces levels of circulating immune complexes in patients with autoimmune diseases [16]. PGE_1 also protects the gastric mucosa against NSAID induced injury [17] and may enhance healing of gastric ulcers [18]. Thus, PGE_1 has a range of desirable potential therapeutic effects distinct from other PGs. Willis [19] was the first to suggest that PGE_1 therapy might be accomplished by providing the PGE_1 precursors GLA and DGLA. The extremely short half-lives of natural prostaglandins have a purpose: they allow moment-to-moment regulation of cell function in response to external stimuli and internal messengers. Exogenous administration of PGE_1, which may be useful in the short-term [15, 16], cannot mimic the physiological variations of endogenous PGE_1. Enrichment of cells with DGLA might enable PGE_1 concentrations to be altered as needed without overriding the physiological controls that modulate rapid changes in its synthesis and degradation. Although it was originally thought that these fatty acids exerted their beneficial effects mainly through modification of the eicosanoid profile and generation of less

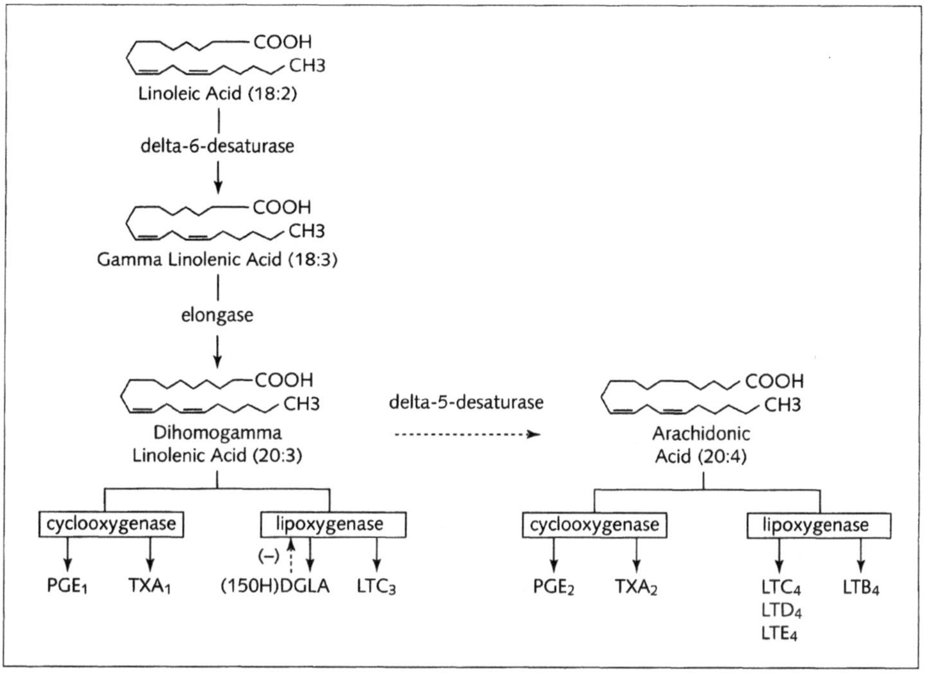

Figure 1
Metabolic pathway of n-6 fatty acids. The pathway consists of alternating steps of desaturation (addition of double bonds) and elongation (addition of carbons).
PGE: prostaglandin E; TXA: thromboxane A; LT: leukotriene

potent mediators of inflammation, observations that they also exert direct effects on cells of the immune system have implications for treatment of RA patients.

Some plant seed oils, notably those extracted from the seeds of *oenethera biennis* (evening primrose) and *boragio officianalis* (borage) contain relatively large amounts of GLA. As noted, GLA is converted to DGLA, the immediate precursor of PGE_1, an eicosanoid with known antiinflammatory and immunoregulating properties [12]. Administration of GLA to volunteers and to RA patients results in increased production of PGE_1 and reduced production of the inflammatory eicosanoids PGE_2, leukotriene B_4 (LTB_4), and LTC_4 by stimulated peripheral blood monocytes [20]. In addition to competing with arachidonic acid for oxidative enzymes, DGLA cannot be converted to inflammatory leukotrienes [21]. Rather, it is converted via 15 lipoxygenase to a 15 hydroxy DGLA which has the capacity to inhibit 5- and 12-lipoxygenase activities [22]. DGLA should therefore have antiinflammatory actions due to its capacity to reduce synthesis of oxygenation products of AA through both the cyclooxygenase and lipoxygenase pathways.

In addition to their role as precursors of eicosanoids, essential fatty acids are important for the maintenance of cell membrane structure and function. DGLA can also modulate immune responses in a prostaglandin independent manner by acting directly on T lymphocytes. For example, DGLA suppresses interleukin-2 (IL-2) production by human peripheral blood mononuclear cells (PBMC) *in vitro*, suppresses proliferation of IL-2 dependent human T lymphocytes, and reduces expression of activation markers on T lymphocytes directly, in a manner which is independent of its conversion to eicosanoids. These actions of GLA are important given the fact that T cell activation appears to be central to propagation of joint tissue injury in RA patients [23].

What appears to be unique about RA is proliferation of synovial cells which line the joint space. The synovial pannus found in the joints of patients with RA is an inflammatory and invasive aggregation of connective tissue, small blood vessels, hyperplastic synovial cells, lymphocytes, plasma cells, and macrophages [24]. It is much like a non-metastatic tumor, and is likely responsible in large part for the cartilage degradation, bone erosion, and irreversible destruction of joints which plague many RA patients. The cause of RA is unknown, and the reasons why cells invade the synovium and why synovial cells proliferate in RA patients have not been defined. Experimental evidence does indicate that products exported by monocytes, macrophages, lymphocytes, and platelets help regulate synovial cell proliferation [24].

Synovial fibroblasts from RA patients have some characteristics similar to cells which have been exposed to tumor promoting agents. Combined epidemiological and experimental evidence supports the importance of fatty acids in tumor growth, although the precise relationships are not clear. Thus, fatty acids and eicosanoids have varying effects *in vitro* and in animals depending on the doses used and the tumor type studied. Plasminogen activator levels are increased in synovial fluid from RA patients compared to patients with osteoarthritis [25], and IL-1 induces plasminogen activator expression in synovial fibroblasts [26]. Connective tissues express plasminogen activator and plasminogen activator inhibitor normally, probably to regulate matrix turnover. It is possible that in RA, increased action of plasminogen activator shifts the balance to degradation by pannus of cartilage and bone. Furthermore, maintenance of the synovial pannus in RA patients, like tumor growth, depends on establishment of new blood vessels and angiogenesis is stimulated by plasminogen activation. Thus, the observation [27] that DGLA and docosahexaenoic acid (DHA; 22:6*n*-3, a major component of fish oil) selectively increase steady state mRNA levels of plasminogen activator inhibitor-1 in human endothelial cells in culture may be potentially important. Addition of DGLA to human synovial cells in culture reduces PGE_2, increases PGE_1, and restrains IL-1 stimulated synovial cell growth [13]. The antiproliferative effect of DGLA is prevented in large part by indomethacin addition to cells. However, as noted, fatty acids themselves, exclusive of their eicosanoid metabolites, are able to influence cell function. Examination of the effects of GLA and DGLA on the function of cells which invade the synovial pannus has yielded important information.

Effects of fatty acids on lymphocyte function

Joint tissue injury in RA patients appears due in large part to activation of T lymphocytes in the synovium [23]. In antigen stimulated T lymphocytes, the complex of T cell antigen receptor (TCR) and CD3, and the CD4 and CD8 proteins physically associate with, and thereby activate, several intracellular protein tyrosine kinases. Tyrosine phosphorylation of phospholipase $C_{\gamma 1}$ ($PLC_{\gamma 1}$) activates this enzyme and initiates the hydrolysis of phosphatidylinositol 4,5, bisphosphate and the generation of inositol 1,4,5 triphosphate (IP_3) and diacyglycerol (DAG). IP_3 in turn mobilizes ionized calcium from bound intracellular stores, whereas DAG in the presence of increased cytosolic free calcium binds to and activates protein kinase C (PKC), a family of serine threonine kinases. These events have been causally related to a variety of responses, of which the best characterized is the transcriptional induction of the IL-2 gene in T cells. IL-2 triggers the activation of a variety of kinases, events which lead to the expression of several DNA binding proteins and to progression of the cell cycle. It has been thought that specific fatty acids may exert their inhibitory effects on lymphocyte function by altering transduction of signals from the plasma membrane to the nucleus after their incorporation and esterification into plasma membrane phospholipids, or perhaps by direct effects of the free fatty acids. Iverson et al. [28] studied the effects of DGLA on arachidonic acid metabolism using mixed cell suspensions of lymphocytes and monocytes *in vitro*; these cells contain both cyclooxygenase and lipoxygenase activity. DGLA at concentrations of 50 and 100 µM (16.5 and 33 µg/ml) reduced LTB_4 formation by 60%. Dose-dependent increases in cyclooxygenase and 15 lipoxygenase products (PGE_1 and 15-hydroxy-eicosatetraenoic (HETE) respectively) were also observed. To determine whether the effect of DGLA on AA conversion to LTB_4 might be mediated via 15-HETE, cells were incubated in the presence of a range of concentrations of 15-HETE; a dose-dependent reduction of LTB_4 production was seen. These results suggest that DGLA and its 15 lipoxygenase metabolite, 15-HETE, selectively inhibit the 5-lipoxygenase pathway and subsequent LTB_4 production.

Several unsaturated fatty acids alter human peripheral blood lymphocyte responses to mitogens. Kelly and Parker [29] showed that low concentrations (0.1–1.0 µg/ml) of LA, GLA, DGLA, and AA stimulate proliferative responses of peripheral blood lymphocytes to mitogen lectins, whereas higher concentrations (more than 10 µg/ml) are inhibitory. The precise mechanisms whereby fatty acids suppress lymphocyte proliferation are not known. The effect was originally thought to be related to their metabolism to PGE compounds, which do suppress mitogenesis. However, addition of DGLA *in vitro* suppresses IL-2 driven proliferation of peripheral blood and synovial compartment T lymphocytes in an eicosanoid independent manner [30, 31]. Experiments with the IL-2 dependent murine T cell line CTL.L2 indicate that only DGLA – selectively among eicosanoid precursors – reduces T cell proliferation [32]. The effect is not reversed by inhibitors of cycloxygenase and lipoxygenase. Experiments suggested indirectly that DGLA influences T cell proliferation by modification of PKC activity [32]. It was then shown [33] that GLA and DGLA *in vitro* suppress total PKC activity but enhance translocation of PKC from cytosol to membrane in human peripheral blood T lymphocytes stimulated with phorbol 12 myristate 13-acetate (PMA). AA and LA do not influence total PKC activity, and have more modest effects than GLA and DGLA on PKC translocation. Alpha linolenic acid, eicosapentaenoic acid (EPA), and palmitic acid do not alter PKC activity or translocation in PMA stimulated cells. That DGLA effects differ somewhat from GLA effects reinforces our growing awareness that these two fatty acids do not necessarily have similar actions, and that GLA/DGLA ratios in cells may be important to cell function. It is not known whether the unique effects of GLA and DGLA are due to effects on PKC isozymes which are different from other fatty acids.

GLA and DGLA, but not EPA, suppress CD3 mediated increases in IP_3 and intracellular calcium in T cells [34]. Thus, the fatty acid effects appear to be exerted early in the signal transduction cascade. Activation of protein tyrosine kinases appears to be the most proximal biochemical event after engagement of the T cell receptor, and phospholipase $C_{\gamma 1}$ (PLC) itself must be tyrosine phosphorylated in order to be activated [35]. GLA added to cells *in vitro* or administered to normal volunteers *in vivo* increases tyrosine phosphorylation of PLC modestly in resting T cells, but suppresses phosphorylation of PLC substantially in cells stimulated with monoclonal antibodies to CD3/CD4 [36]. T cell proliferation is also reduced after oral administration of GLA in capsules of borage seed oil. Oral administration of oils enriched in linoleic acid, the parent *n*-6 fatty acid, and α-linolenic acid, the parent *n*-3 fatty acid, does not influence growth of stimulated cells. Fatty acid analyses indicate that suppression of lymphocyte proliferation after GLA administration is associated with increased plasma and PBMC concentrations of GLA and DGLA. Further, the analyses suggest that conversion of GLA to DGLA is necessary for maximum suppression of T lymphocyte activation [36].

Stimulation of lymphocytes through the TCR causes redistribution of cell surface proteins including clustering of the complex of TCR and CD3 with CD4, which with other proteins functions as a unit to initiate T cell activation [37]. Fatty acids constitute an important component of the cell membrane structure and confer on membranes properties of fluidity and flexibility that are key determinants of receptor expression and of protein movement in the membrane [38]. Unsaturated fatty acids disorder the membrane interior and order the head group region [39]; saturated fatty acids do not perturb acyl chain packing, and therefore have less effect on membrane function. A new acyl chain arrangement resulting from administration of

GLA might alter movement of membrane proteins that regulate cell responses. It is likely that perturbation of acyl chain order alters the interaction between membrane lipids and specific proteins, which in turn would alter the function of the proteins [40]. Extremely small changes in membrane fatty acids can influence cell function [41]. Thus, alteration of acyl chain order and suppression of T lymphocyte activation by oral administration of certain unsaturated fatty acids is a distinct possibility, and may help explain why GLA administration does in fact suppress active synovitis in rheumatoid arthritis patients.

Effects on monocyte/macrophage function

As the chief source of IL-1β and TNFα, monocytes are critical to regulation of pathological processes that lead to chronic inflammation and tissue injury. Addition of DGLA *in vitro* and administration of GLA *in vivo* reduces both IL-1β and TNFα production by stimulated human peripheral blood monocytes [36]. GLA administration to normal volunteers and to RA patients increases monocyte production of PGE_1 and reduces production of LTB_4 [20]. The ratio of DGLA to AA in circulating mononuclear cells after administration of GLA increases significantly in both healthy subjects and RA patients.

Effects on platelet function

The extraordinary rapidity with which platelets adhere to damaged tissue, aggregate, and release potent biologically active materials suggests that they may function as a cellular trigger for the inflammatory process. It is generally believed that GLA and DGLA administration decrease platelet aggregation, most likely by a PGE_1-mediated process. Kernoff et al. [42] gave DGLA (0.1–2.0 g) to healthy subjects as a single dose or daily for periods up to 1 month. DGLA consistently reduced platelet aggregation, an effect that was more pronounced with sustained treatment. Using platelet-rich plasma, the investigators found increased production of PGE_1. Unexplained is the finding of an increased capacity of platelets to produce PGE_2, which occurred without evidence of appreciable conversion of DGLA to AA, the biosynthetic precursor of PGE_2. Barre et al. [43] gave a very large dose of GLA (5.23 g/day) in the form of borage seed oil for 6 weeks to healthy male subjects and found increased aggregation of washed platelet suspensions after 3 and 6 weeks of borage seed oil supplementation. Unexpectedly, production by platelets of PGE_1, PGE_2, and TXA_2 did not change during the entire study or during the recovery phase. Siess et al. [44] found that DGLA added to suspensions of washed human platelets, but not to platelet-rich plasma, caused platelet activation as determined by platelet shape change and activation of phospholipase C. Thus, the surprising finding that borage seed oil enhances platelet aggregation may relate to the use of washed rather than unwashed platelets. Also, the dose of GLA given in the Barre study was very high, a critical point, considering the observations of Navarette et al. [45] who found, in guinea pigs, that low-dose GLA increased tissue levels of DGLA but very high doses of GLA decreased epidermal levels of DGLA. The investigators attribute the findings to suppressed conversion by tissue microsomal elongase of GLA to DGLA and suggest that microsomal elongase is regulated in a biphasic manner by its fatty acid substrate, GLA.

Effects on neutrophil function

LTB_4 formation by human neutrophils is suppressed in a dose-dependent manner by both DGLA and LA [46]. At the highest concentrations of fatty acids tested (100 μM = 33 μg/mL), DGLA resulted in 85% reduction of LTB_4 formation, whereas LA reduced LTB_4 by 60%. A concomitant increase in the 15-lipoxygenase (LO) products of DGLA (15-HETE) and LA (13-hydroxy-octadecadienoic acid) was found. Both of these metabolites directly inhibit LTB_4 synthesis by neutrophils. Saturated fatty acids do not influence LTB4 formation.

GLA reduced neutrophil chemotaxis in an animal model; neutrophils isolated from rats fed 65 mg/day GLA in the form of evening primrose oil for 2 weeks showed a greater than 60% reduction in chemotaxis compared with controls [47]. Tate et al. [48] showed that administration of GLA for 24 days suppressed the cellular phase of acute inflammation, which is characterized by neutrophil invasion, in the rat subcutaneous air pouch model.

Studies in animal models

GLA suppresses acute and chronic inflammation including joint injury in several experimental animal models. In animals treated with evening primrose or borage seed oils, cells from inflammatory exudate are enriched in GLA and DGLA, exudate PGE_2 and LTB_4 are reduced [48], and leucocyte effector function (chemotaxis, lysosomal enzyme release) is suppressed [47]. It is interesting to note that in the rat subcutaneous air pouch model, GLA treatment suppressed the cellular phase (neutrophil invasion, pouch lining proliferation) but had little effect on the fluid phase (exudate volume, protein concentration) of acute inflammation. In contrast, fish oil reduced the exudate volume and protein concentration substantially, but it did not influence neutrophil invasion, neutrophil function, or lining cell proliferation. The findings indicate that the fluid and cellular phases of the acute inflammatory response can be regulated independently. They suggest further that adequate control of these separate events might require therapy with more than one agent. In fact, a combination of fish oil and primrose seed oil supplements reduced both the cellular and fluid phases of monosodium urate crystal-induced inflammation [48]. In addition, the tissue DGLA to AA ratio is increased substantially in animals fed a combination diet enriched in both GLA and EPA. The increase probably results from inhibition by EPA of the conversion of DGLA to AA [49].

Clinical trials

A placebo-controlled study [50] indicated that 20 patients given GLA (360 mg/day) in the form of primrose seed oil for 12 weeks received no benefits from such therapy. It is of interest that although only 3 patients improved clinically, all but 2 of the remaining patients were able to complete the study without resorting to other NSAIDs. Thus, although the study was considered to be "negative", the results suggest that GLA might substitute for NSAID treatment. In a double-blind, placebo-controlled study [51], 16 patients with RA received 540 mg/day of GLA as primrose seed oil and 15 patients received 450 mg/day GLA and 240 mg/day of EPA for one year. Patients were kept on their usual dose of NSAIDs, and their physicians were allowed to alter the dose according to clinical responses. Patients did not exhibit changes in objective measures of their disease activity, but over 90% of patients in the treatment group felt subjective improvement in their condition at 12 months at which time 50% of treated patients had either stopped or reduced substantially the NSAID dose. In a study [52] designed to investigate the effect of GLA on leukocyte function, PGE_2 and LTB_4 production by stimulated leukocytes was reduced markedly, and 6 of 7 RA patients appeared to respond favorably over a 12 week period to treatment with 1.1 gm/day GLA in the form of borage seed oil; the study was not placebo-controlled. Unlike the other studies with smaller doses of GLA, RA patients given borage seed oil did exhibit reductions in the duration of painful morning stiffness and the number of tender swollen joints. Brzeski et al. [53] did a 6 month study of 40 patients with RA who had evidence (endoscopic, radiographic, or clinical symptoms) suggestive of upper gastrointestinal lesions, presumably caused by NSAID use. The aim of the study was to determine whether patients given GLA would experience enough improvement in joint symptoms to allow reduction of the NSAID dose. Patients were given either 540 mg GLA per day or 6 gm per day of olive oil. Morning stiffness was reduced significantly at both 3 and 6 months in the GLA group, and a reduction in pain and articular index at 6 months was seen in patients given olive oil. However, only 23% of the patients in the GLA group and 18% of patients in the olive oil group were able to reduce their NSAID dose. Although patients in this study had more severe RA than patients in the earlier study [51], none were treated with second line drugs. Beneficial effects of olive oil in RA have been reported [54]. Therefore, olive oil can no longer be considered an inert placebo. Also, individual variations in levels of $\Delta 5$ desaturase may alter the response to GLA. It is generally believed that humans have low levels of this enzyme and hence limited conversion of DGLA to AA. However, a small but significant increase in serum arachidonate was reported in one group of RA patients who took 1.8 gm/day GLA for 3 months [8]. Reduced plasma PGE_2 in these patients was associated with a good therapeutic response to GLA.

GLA treatment of RA was evaluated in a 24 week randomized, double-blind, placebo-controlled (cotton seed oil) trial [55]. Only patients with RA on a stable NSAID and/or low corticosteroid dose (<10 mg/day prednisone or equivalent) that was continued through the study period were allowed to participate. Treatment with GLA (1.4 gm/day in borage seed oil) resulted in clinically important reductions in signs and symptoms of disease activity. In contrast, patients given placebo showed no change or worsening of disease. GLA reduced the number of tender joints by 36%, tender joint score by 45%, swollen joint count by 28%, and swollen joint score by 41%, whereas the placebo group did not show significant improvement in any measure. Overall clinical responses (more than 25% improvement in four measures) were also significantly better in the treatment group. Platelet counts were reduced significantly in the GLA group but neither erythrocyte sedimentation rate nor rheumatoid factor changed appreciably in either group. In a larger study [56], 56 patients with active RA were randomized to treatment groups in a 6 month double-blind trial of GLA versus placebo, followed by a 6 month single-blind trial during which all patients received GLA. Patients were treated with 2.8 gm/day of GLA as the free fatty acid or with sunflower seed oil administered in identical capsules. Treatment with GLA for 6 months resulted in statistically significant and clinically relevant reductions in the signs and symptoms of disease activity in patients with RA. Overall meaningful responses were also better in the GLA treatment group (14 of 22 patients versus 4 of 19 in the placebo groups; $p = 0.015$). During the second 6 months, both groups exhibited improvement in disease activity. Thus, patients taking GLA during the entire study showed progressive improvement during the second 6 months. In this group, 16 of 21 patients showed meaningful improvement at 12 months compared with study entry. Thus, GLA at doses used in this study is a well tolerated and effective treatment for active RA. GLA is available as a component of several plant seed oils, and is usually taken in far lower doses than were used in this last trial. It is not approved in the United States for the treatment of any condition, and should not be viewed as therapy for any disease. Although adverse effects of GLA administration have been negligible (mainly belching, abdomial bloating, loose stools in an occasional patient), potential problems cannot be dismissed. Administration of long chain polyunsaturated fatty acids increases the likelihood of lipid peroxidation with its associated toxic effects on cells. It is not known whether an increased requirement for antioxidants such as vitamins E and C accompanies increased intake of GLA. We have considered, and others have shown in a controlled clinical trial [51], that GLA can be an NSAID substitute. However, our observations that DGLA suppresses synovial cell proliferation [13], and the results of the study [56] which indicated that RA patients are better after 12 months of GLA treatment than after 6 months, suggest that GLA might function as a so-called DMARD (disease modifying anti-rheumatic drug). Thus, controlled studies of longer duration on larger numbers of RA patients in which GLA is compared with more established "second line therapy", and which use radiographs to monitor disease progression are warranted.

Fatty acid analysis of plasma or circulating cells was not used as a measure of compliance in these studies because the amount of GLA or DGLA present after administration of a known amount of GLA varies from person to person, and would not necessarily reflect the number of capsules of GLA ingested. However, it is important to know that plasma and cell concentrations of GLA and/or DGLA during GLA therapy can reach levels equivalent to concentrations of fatty acids which *in vitro* suppress lymphocyte activation and synovial cell proliferation. Plasma levels of GLA and DGLA were increased two to four-fold in the GLA treated patients to concentrations which exceed those needed to exert effects *in vitro* [56]. Similarly, concentrations of GLA and DGLA in platelets increased as much as eightfold during GLA treatment. Lower doses of GLA used in previous studies (480 to 540 mg/day) were either not effective or reduced only pain without effects on physical findings. In controlled clinical trials in which GLA was shown to benefit patients with atopic eczema [57], some patients responded very well, others modestly. Clinical responses seemed to correlate with plasma levels of DGLA. Indeed, in a study in which benefit from GLA was not observed [58], plasma levels of DGLA did not rise. Thus, responses to GLA do appear to be dose-dependent.

The potential regulation of cell activation, immune responses, and inflammation by unsaturated fatty acids is exciting to consider at the clinical, cellular, and molecular levels. A better understanding of how fatty acids modulate function of cells involved in host defense might lead to development of new, benign treatment for diseases such as rheumatoid arthritis that are characterized by acute and chronic inflammation.

References

1 Wolfe AM (1968) The epidemiology of rheumatoid arthritis. A review. *Bull Rheum Dis* 19: 518–532

2 Gran JT (1987) The epidemiology of rheumatoid arthritis. *Monogr Allergy* 21: 162–196

3 Silman AJ, MacGregor AJ, Thomson W (1993) Twin concordance rates for rheumatoid arthritis: A nationwide study. *Br J Rheumatol* 32: 903–912

4 MacGregor A, Ollier W, Thompson W, Jawaheer D, Silman A (1995) HLA-DRB1 0401/0404 genotype and rheumatoid arthritis: Increased association in men, young age at onset, and disease severity. *J Rheumatol* 22: 1030–1036

5 Pincus T, Brooks RH, Callahan LF (1994) Prediction of long-term mortality in patients

with rheumatoid arthritis according to simple questionnaire and joint count measures. *Annals Int Med* 120: 26–34
6 Horrobin DF, Manku MS (1990) Clinical biochemistry of essential fatty acids. In: DF Horrobin (ed): *Omega-6 essential fatty acids. Pathophysiology and roles in clinical medicine.* Wiley-Liss, New York, 21–53
7 Danon A, Heimberg M, Oates JA (1975) Enrichment of rat tissue lipids with fatty acids that are prostaglandin precursors. *Biochim Biophys Acta* 388: 318–330
8 Jantti J, Nikkari T, Solakivi T (1989) Evening primrose oil in rheumatoid arthritis: Changes in serum lipids and fatty acids. *Ann Rheum Dis* 48: 124–127
9 van Dorp DA, Beerthuis RK, Nugteren DH (1964) The biosynthesis of prostaglandins. *Biochem Biophys Acta* 90: 204–207
10 Bergstrom S, Daniellson H, Samuelsson B (1964) The enzymatic formation of prostaglandin E_2 from arachadonic acid. *Biochem Biophys Acta* 90: 207–210
11 Bergstrom S, Daniellson H, Klenberg D, Samuelsson B (1964) The enzymatic conversion of essential fatty acids into prostaglandins. *J Biol Chem* 239: 4006–4008
12 Zurier RB (1990) Prostaglandin E_1: Is it useful? (editorial) *J Rheumatol* 17: 1439–1441
13 Baker DG, Krakauer KA, Tate G, Zurier RB (1989) Suppression of human synovial cell proliferation by dihomogammalinolenic acid. *Arth Rheumatol* 32: 1273–1281
14 Pelletier J, Dibattista JA, Ranger P (1994) The reduced expression of glucocorticoid receptors in synovial cells induced by nonsteroidal antiinflammatory drugs can be reversed by a prostaglandin E_1 analog. *J Rheumatol* 21: 1748–1742
15 Fantone JC, Kunkel SL, Ward PA, Zurier RB (1981) Suppression of human polymorphonuclear function after intravenous infusion of prostaglandin E_1. *Prostaglandins Med* 7: 195–198
16 Yoshikawa T, Sukuki H, Kato H (1990) Effects of prostaglandin E1 on collagen diseases with high levels of circulating immune complexes. *J Rheumatol* 17: 1513–1514
17 Graham DY, White RH, Moreland LW (1993) Duodenal and gastric ulcer prevention with misoprostol in arthritis patients taking NSAIDs. *Ann Int Med* 119: 257–262
18 Walt RP (1992) Misoprostol for the treatment of peptic ulcer and antiinflammatory drug induced gastroduodenal ulceration. *N Engl J Med* 327: 1575–1580
19 Willis AL (1981) Nutritional and pharmacological factors in eicosanoid biology. *Nutr Rev* 39: 289–301
20 Callegari PE, Zurier RB (1991) Botanical lipids: Potential role in modulation of immunologic responses and inflammatory reactions. *Rheum Dis Clin NA* 17: 415–425
21 Hammarstrom S (1981) Conversion of dihomogammalinolenic acid to an isomer of leukotriene C_3 oxygenated at C-8. *J Biol Chem* 256: 7712–7714
22 Ziboh VA, Chapkin RS (1987) Biologic significance of polyunsaturated fatty acids in the skin. *Arch Dermatol* 123: 1686–1690
23 Panayi GS (1993) The immunopathogenesis of rheumatoid arthritis. *Br J Rheum* 32 (suppl 1): 4–14
24 Harris ED, Jr (1997) *Rheumatoid arthritis.* WB Saunders Company, Philadelphia

25 Mochan E, Uhl J (1994) Elevations in synovial fluid plasminogen activator in patients with rheumatoid arthritis. *J Rheumatol* 11: 123–128

26 Mochan E, Uhl J, Newton R (1986) Interleukin-1 stimulation of synovial cell plasminogen activator production. *J Rheumatol* 13: 15–19

27 Kariko K, Rosenbaum H, Kuo A, Zurier RB, Barnathan ES (1995) Stimulatory effect of unsaturated fatty acids on the level of plasminogen activator inhibitor-1 mRNA in cultured human endothelial cells. *FEBS Lett* 361: 118–122

28 Iverson L, Fogh K, Kragbelle K (1992) Effect of dihomogammalinolenic acid and its 15 lipoxygenase metabolite on eicosanoid metabolism by human mononuclear leukocytes *in vitro*: Selective inhibition of the 5 lipoxygenase pathway. *Arch Dermatol Res* 284: 222–226

29 Kelly JP, Parker CW (1979) Effects of arachadonic acid and other unsaturated fatty acids on mitogenesis in human lymphocytes. *J Immunol* 122: 1556–1562

30 Santoli D, Phillips PD, Colt TL, Zurier RB (1990) Suppression of interleukin-2 dependent human T cell growth *in vitro* by prostaglandin E and their precursor fatty acids: Evidence for a PGE independent mechanism of inhibition by the fatty acids. *J Clin Invest* 85: 424–432

31 DeMarco DM, Santoli D, Zurier RB (1994) Effects of fatty acids on proliferation and activation of human synovial compartment lymphocytes. *J Leuk Biol* 56: 612–615

32 Borofsky MA, Zurier RB, Rosenbaum H, Williams WV (1992) Effects of polyunsaturated fatty acids on interleukin-2 dependent T cell growth. *Immunol Res* 11: 154–164

33 Rossetti RG, Seiler CM, Laposata M, Zurier RB (1995) Differential regulation of human T lymphocyte protein kinase C activity by unsaturated fatty acids. *Clin Immunol Immunopathol* 76: 220–224

34 Vassilopoulos D, Zurier RB, Rossetti RG, Tsokos GC (1997) Gammalinolenic acid in dihomogammalinolenic acid suppressed the CD3 mediated signal transduction pathway in human T cells. *Clin Immunol Immunopathol* 83: 237–244

35 June CH, Fletcher MC, Ledbetter JA, Samelson LE (1990) Increases in tyrosine phosphorylation are detectable before phospholipase C activation after T cell receptor stimulation. J Immunol 144:1591–1597

36 Rossetti RG, DeLuca P, Seiler CM, Zurier AW, Karim P, Zurier RB (1997) Modification of human lymphocyte and monocyte function by gammalinolenic acid, an unsaturated fatty acid: Studies *in vitro* and *in vivo*. *Arthritis Rheum* 40: S177

37 Miceli MC, Parnes JR (1991) The roles of CD4 and CD3 in T cell activation. *Sem Immunol* 3: 133–147

38 McMurchie EJ (1988) Dietary lipids and the regulation of membrane fluidity and function. In: RC Aloia (eds): *Physiological regulation of membrane fluidity*. Liss, New York, 189–204

39 Klausner RD, Kleinfeld AM, Hoover RL, Karnovsky ML (1980) Lipid domains in membranes: Evidence derived from structural perturbations induced by free fatty acids and life-time heterogeneity analysis. *J Biol Chem* 255: 1286–1290

40 Anel A, Richieri GV, Kleinfeld AM (1993) Membrane partition of fatty acids and inhibition of T cell function. *Biochem* 32: 530–534

41 Richieri GV, Kleinfeld AM (1989) Free fatty acid perturbation of transmembrane signaling in cytotoxic T lymphocytes. *J Immunol* 143: 2302–2307

42 Kernoff PBA, Willis AL, Stone KJ, Davies JA, McNichol GP (1977) Antithrombotic potential of dihomogammalinolenic acid. *Br Med J* 2: 1441–1444

43 Barre DE, Holub BJ, Chapkin RS (1993) The effect of borage oil supplementation on human platelet aggregation, thromboxing B2, prostaglandin E_1 and E_2 formation. *Nutr Res* 13: 739–751

44 Siess W, Siegel FL, Lapetina EG (1984) Dihomogammalinolenic acid, but not eicosapenteoic acid, activates washed human platelets. *Biochem Biophys Acta* 801: 265–276

45 Navarette R, Tang W, Ziboh VA (1992) Dietary intake of concentrated gammalinolenic acid (GLA) enriched oil suppresses cutaneous level of dihomogammalinolenic acid (DGLA): Possible *in vivo* inhibition of microsomelongation of GLA to DGLA. *Prostaglandins Leukot Essent Fatty Acids* 46: 139–144

46 Iverson L, Fogh K, Bojesen G (1991) Linoleic acid and dihomogammalinolenic acid inhibit leukotriene formation and stimulate the formation of their 15 lipoxygenase products by human neutrophils *in vitro*. Evidence of formation of antiinflammatory compounds. *Agents Actions* 33: 286–291

47 Kunkel SL, Ogawa H, Ward, PA, Zurier RB (1981) Suppression of chronic inflammation by evening primrose oil. *Prog Lipid Res* 20: 885–888

48 Tate GA, Mandell BF, Karmali RA, Laposata M, Baker DG, Schumacher HR, Zurier RB (1988) Suppression of monosodium murate crystal induced acute inflammation by diets enriched with gammalinolenic acid and eicosapentenoic acid. *Arthritis Rheum* 31: 1543–1551

49 Needleman P, Raz A, Minkes NS (1979) Triene prostaglandins: Prostacyclin and thromboxane biosynthesis and unique biological properties. *Proc Natl Acad Sci USA* 76: 940–949

50 Mork-Hansen T, Lerche A, Kassis V, Lorenzen I, Sondergaard J (1983) Treatment of rheumatoid arthritis with prostaglandin E_2 precursors cis-linoleic acid and gammalinolenic acid. *Scand J Rheum* 12: 85–88

51 Belch JJF, Madhok AR, OíDowd A, Sturrock RD (1988) Effects of altering dietary essential fatty acids on requirements for nonsteroidal antiinflammatory drugs in patients with rheumatoid arthritis: A double blind placebo controlled study. *Ann Rheum Dis* 47: 96–104

52 Pullman-Moar SW, Laposata M, Lem D, Holman RT, Leventhal LJ, DeMarco D, Zurier RB (1990) Alteration of the cellular fatty acid profile and the production of eicosanoids in human monocytes by gammalinolenic acid. *Arthritis Rheum* 33: 1526–1534

53 Brezeski M, Madhok R, Capell HA (1991) Evening primrose oil in patients with rheumatoid arthritis and side effects of non-steroidal antiinflammatory drugs. *Br J Rheum* 30: 370–372

54 Darlington LG, Ramsey NW (1987) Olive oil for rheumatoid patients? *Br J Rheum* 26 (suppl 2): 129
55 Leventhal LJ, Boyce EG, Zurier RB (1993) Treatment of rheumatoid arthritis with gammalinolenic acid. *Ann Int Med* 119: 867–873
56 Zurier RB, Rossetti RG, Jacobson, EW, DeMarco DM, Liu NY, Temming JE, White BM, Laposata M (1996) Gammalinolenic acid treatment of rheumatoid arthritis. A randomized, placebo-controlled trial. *Arthritis Rheum* 39: 1808–1817
57 Wright S, Burton JL (1982) Oral evening primrose oil improves atopic eczema. *Lancet* 2: 1120–1122
58 Bamford JT, Gibson RW, Renier CM (1985) Atopic eczema unresponsive to evening primrose oil (linoleic and gammalinolenic acids). *J Acad Dermatol* 13: 959–965

59. Darlington C, Stinson [illegible] (199[illegible]) [illegible] [illegible]

[illegible] [illegible] gammahydroxybutyric acid. Am J Psychiatry 149: [illegible]

58. Zand KS, Lucero RG, [illegible] [illegible] (19[illegible]) [illegible] 11, 57 [illegible]

[illegible]

[illegible]

The role of *n*-3 fatty acids in psoriasis

Vincent A. Ziboh

Department of Dermatology, University of California, Davis, Davis, CA 95616, USA

Introduction

In 1929, Burr and Burr [1] presented the first in a series of papers outling a "new deficiency disease produced by the rigid exclusion of fat from the diet." They developed the hypothesis that warm-blooded animals cannot synthesize appreciable quantities of certain fatty acids. In 1930 both investigators significantly added to their earlier work by presenting evidence that the dietary inclusion of linoleic acid alone could reverse all deficiency symptoms resulting from a fat-free diet and thus linoleic acid (LA or 18:2*n*-6) was heralded as an "essential fatty acid" (EFA) [2]. [Fatty acids and acyl groups are denoted 18:2*n*-6, 18:3*n*-3 and so on, with the first number representing the number of carbons in the acyl chain, the number following the colon indicating the number of methylene interrupted cis-double bonds and the number of "*n*" indicating the number of carbon atoms from the methyl end of the acyl chain to the nearest double bond.] This pioneering study contained additional observations which indicated that besides the visible scaliness of the skin, animals with essential fatty acid deficiency (EFAD) also experience increased water consumption without increased urine output leading to speculation of increased water loss through the skin. Thus, Burr recognized in these early studies the two major defects that have been associated with EFA deficiency in cutaneous biology, namely, epidermal hyperproliferation and an increased permeability of the skin to water.

Structural forms

Three major families of unsaturated fatty acids (UFAs) are characteristic of mammalian species; the *n*-9, the *n*-6, and the *n*-3 UFAs. the *n*-6 and *n*-3 polyunsaturated fatty acids (PUFAs) are defined by the position of the double bond closest to the terminal methyl group of the fatty acid molecule. For instance, in the *n*-6 family, the first double bond occurs between the sixth and seventh carbons from the methyl group end of the molecule, whereas in the *n*-3 family the first double bond occurs

Medicinal Fatty Acids in Inflammation, edited by J. Kremer

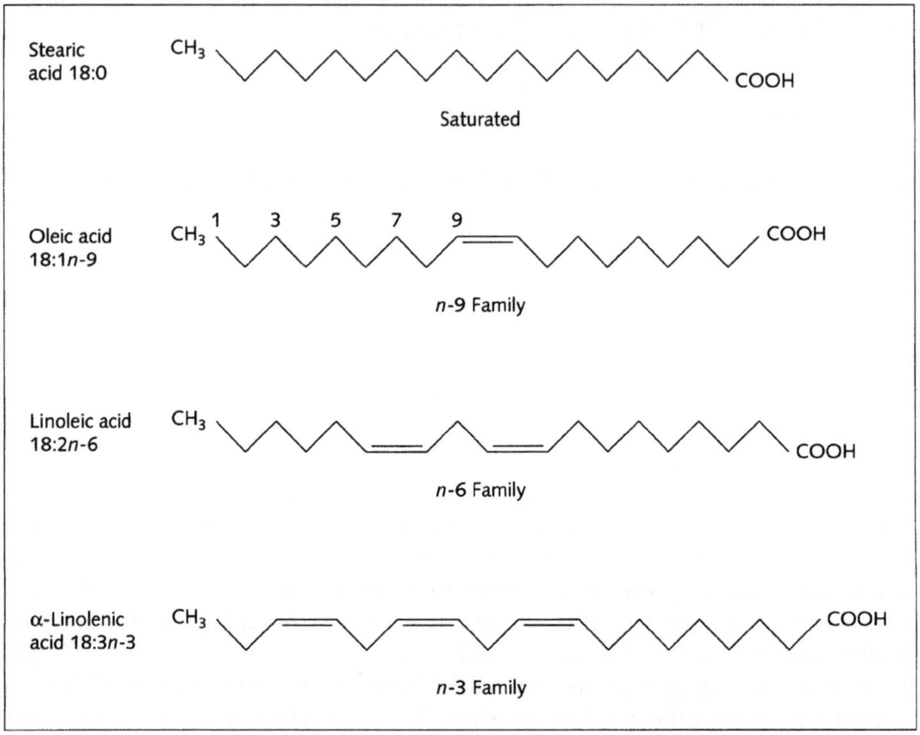

Figure 1
*Representative structures of 18-carbon: saturated (stearic acid, 18:0), monounsaturated (oleic acid, 18:1*n*-9), diunsaturated (linoleic acid, 18:2*n*-6), and triunsaturated (α-linolenic acid, 18:3*n*-3).*

between the third and fourth carbons. These structural forms are shown in Figure 1. These basic structures cannot be synthesized *de novo* by vertebrate animals nor are the *n*-3 and *n*-6 families of PUFAs interconvertible. Thus, these PUFAs must be obtained from the diet.

Dietary sources

The 18-carbon *n*-6 and *n*-3 polyunsaturated fatty acids (PUFAs) are synthesized on land by many plants and therefore are obtained from vegetable oils. However, the longer chain members of each family are either biosynthesized *in vivo* after dietary ingestion of the shorter 18-carbon precursors or they are obtained directly from animal or marine sources. For example, the longer chain *n*-3 PUFAs, eicosapentaenoic acid (EPA, 20:5*n*-3) and docosahexaenoic acid (DHA, 22:6*n*-3), are found in fish and marine oils and therefore can be ingested directly from these sources.

Metabolism of EFA – desaturation and elongation of shorter chain PUFAs

The shorter chain EFAs, linoleic acid (LA, 18:2*n*-6) and α-linolenic acid (α-LA, 18:3*n*-3), serve as the initial polyunsaturated precursors for the *in vivo* biosynthesis of the longer chain PUFAs. Metabolism of the EFAs in most tissues involves an alternating sequence of Δ^6 desaturation, chain elongation, and Δ^5 desaturation in which two hydrogen atoms are removed to create a new double bond followed by the addition of two carbon atoms to lengthen the fatty acid chain [3] (Fig. 2). The desaturations are catalyzed by two separate enzymes: the Δ^6 desaturase (catalyzing the transformation of 18:2*n*-6 to 18:3*n*-6) and the Δ^5 desaturase (catalyzing the transformation of 20:3*n*-6 to 20:4*n*-6). The elongase enzyme catalyzes the elongation of 18:3*n*-6 to 20:3*n*-6 dihomogammalinolenic acid (DGLA) [3]. It is believed that the same enzymes catalyze equivalent steps in the *n*-3, *n*-6 and *n*-9 pathways [4]. The PUFA families interact in such a manner that the *n*-3 acids competitively suppress the bioconversion of the *n*-6 acids, while the *n*-6 suppress the metabolism of the *n*-3 acids, although less markedly. Both the *n*-6 and the *n*-3 acids suppress the formation of the nonessential long chain *n*-9 acids, hence the negligible formation of the long chain *n*-9 PUFA (20:3*n*-9) in nomally fed animals.

The physiological role of *n*-3 polyunsaturated fatty acids in the skin

The physiological role of the *n*-3 PUFAs in the biology of skin is not completely clear. As a first step, in an attempt to determine whether the *n*-3 PUFAs exert any physiological effect in skin, the diet of normal guinea pigs was supplemented with fish oil containing eicosapentaenoic acid (EPA, 20:5*n*-3) and docosahexaenoic acid (DHA, 22:6*n*-3). An interesting finding is the incorporation of the *n*-3 PUFAs (EPA and DHA) into specific epidermal phospholipids [5]. For instance, dietary EPA is incorporated mainly into epidermal phosphatidylcholine (PC) whereas DHA is incorporated preferentially into phosphatidylethanolamine (PE). The significance of the preferential distributions of these two major *n*-3 PUFAs in fish oil into selected phospholipids and the turnover of these pools of phospholipids remains to be elucidated.

Coincident with the uptake of *n*-3 PUFAs into epidermal phospholipids is the elevation of epidermal levels of 15-hydroxyeicosapentaenoic acid (15-HEPE), an oxidative metabolite of EPA, which is catalyzed by the epidermal 15-lipoxygenase *in vivo*. In contrast to EPA, the epidermal metabolite of DHA (17-hydroxydocosahexaenoic acid, 17-HDoHE) was not detected in the epidermis of these animals,

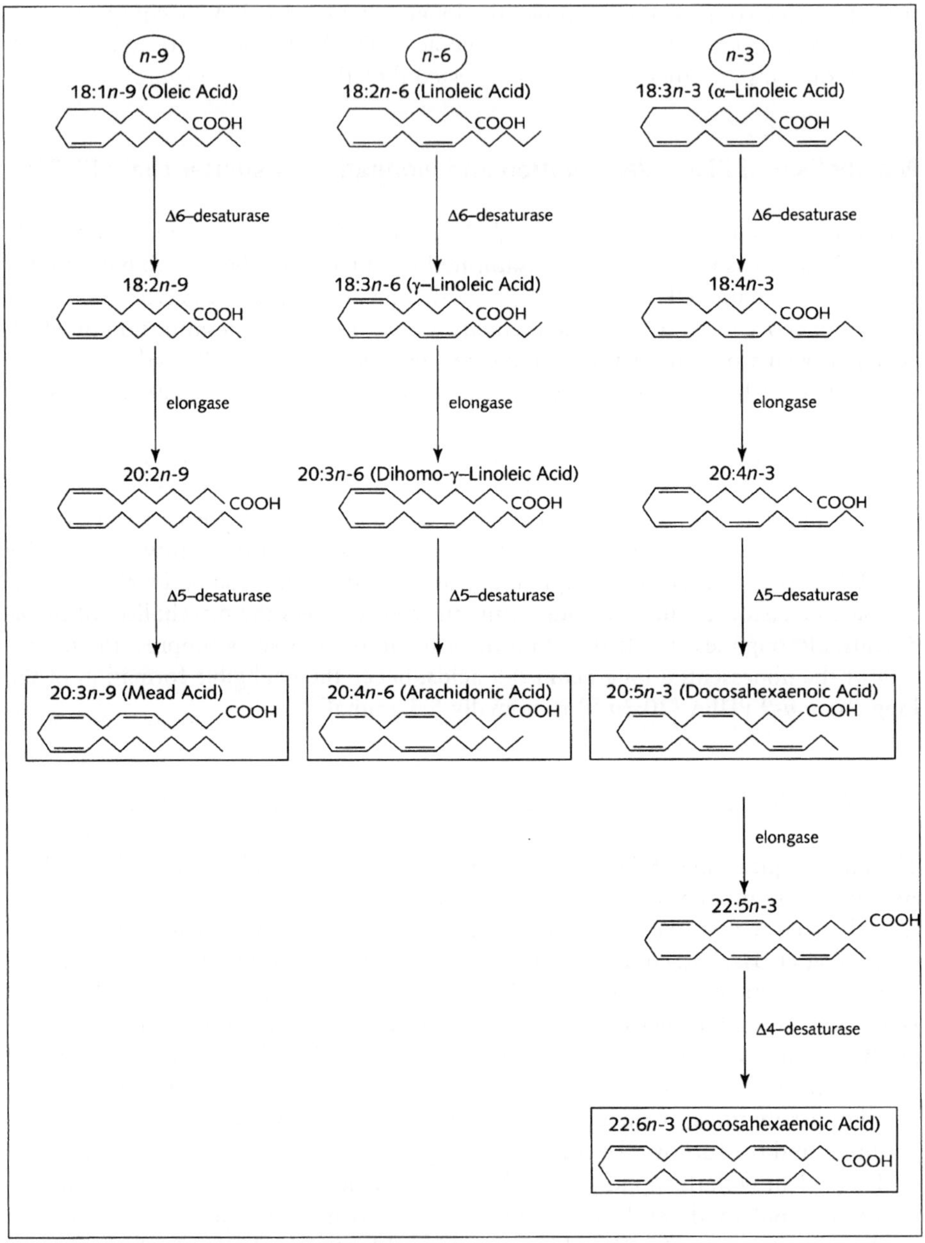

Figure 2
Oxidative desaturation and elongation of n-9, n-6 *and* n-3 *polyunsaturated fatty acids.*

even though DHA was incorporated into the pool of epidermal PE phospholipids. It remains to be established whether DHA is incorporated into alkyl- or alkenyl-acyl ether-linked PEs rather than diacyl PE. This latter observation, nonetheless, suggests that although DHA is incorporated preferentially into a pool of epidermal PE, this pool of phospholipid or its subset, is presumably unavailable to the epidermal phospholipases for hydrolysis and release of DHA for lipoxygenation into 17-HDoHE (a potent *in vitro* inhibitor of 5-lipoxygenase activity). This raises the possibility that multiple forms of phospholipases may exist in the epidermis which hydrolyze fatty acids from selected phospholipid pools.

Dietary role of *n*-3 PUFAs on the clinical course of psoriasis

The possibility that EPA could compete with arachidonic acid (AA) at the substrate level for incorporation into membrane phospholipids, thereby decreasing the metabolism of AA into eicosanoids, prompted us to hypothesize that a diet low in AA, but rich in EPA, could improve the inflammatory/proliferative aspects of psoriasis. Psoriasis is a chronic hyperinflammatory and hyperproliferative skin disorder. The lesions are often infiltrated, scaly and erythematous. Histologically, the lesions are characterized by hyperplasia, incomplete differentiation of the epidermis, dilated capillaries in the papillary dermis and by leukocytes infiltrating both epidermis and dermis. We reasoned that dietary manipulation of polyunsaturated fats which enriched *n*-3 PUFAs, particularly EPA, could result in a significant reduction on both the hyperinflammatory and hyperproliferative components of psoriasis, which are induced by elevated levels of AA proinflammatory lipoxygenase products. The first study of the association of AA and psoriasis was by Hammarstrom et al. [6] who reported elevated levels of free AA, PGE_2, and $PGF_{2\alpha}$ (AA cyclooxygenase products) and 12-hydroxyeicosatetraenoic (HETE) (AA lipoxygenase product). Subsequently, new reports revealed that a leukotriene B_4- (LTB_4-) like material was detected in scale and skin recovered from psoriatic plaques [7–11].

To determine whether diet supplemented with *n*-3 PUFAs would ameliorate the lesions of psoriasis, we tested in an open trial study the efficacy of dietary fish oil (Max-EPA), which is rich in EPA and DHA in a group of eighteen adult patients with stable psoriasis vulgaris. Each patient's diet was supplemented with fish oil which contained approximately: EPA (10.8 g), DHA (7.2 g) and AA (0.6 g) per day. After eight weeks, the clinical findings revealed mild to moderate improvement of their lesions in terms of the scaling, thickness and erythema in approximately 60% of the eighteen patients [12]. The initial beneficial effects reported above were followed by two other dietary studies. For example, in another open trial study [13], the investigators provided fish oil (containing approximately 12 g EPA/day) to ten psoriatic patients for six weeks and reported moderate beneficial effects in 8 patients. Additionally, this group reported a marked suppression of LTB_4 from Ca^{2+} ionophore-activated polymorphonuclear cells (PMNs) isolated from patients. Furthermore, in a double-blind, randomized, placebo-controlled trial study, 28 patients with stable psoriasis received Max-EPA capsules equivalent to 1.8 g EPA/day for 8–12 weeks. After eight weeks, investigators reported a lessening of itching, erythema and scaling in the active treatment group when compared to the placebo group [14]. Thus, in three studies, two open trials and one double blind, the possible beneficial effects of dietary *n*-3 PUFA on the clinical course of psoriasis has been indicated.

However, in another double-blind study, investigators reported that administration of Max-EPA (equivalent to 1.8 g EPA/day) for eight weeks resulted in no statistical difference in clinical manifestations of psoriasis between the active treatment group and the placebo group [15]. The reason for discrepancy in the latter two double-blind studies, both supplementing diets with the same amount of *n*-3 PUFA (1.8 g EPA/day) is not immediately clear. It should be noted however, that in these studies, the content of administered EPA (1.8 g EPA/day) is several-fold less than those used in earlier open trial studies. Secondly, the quality of oils used in the latter two double-blind studies and the population of patients could contribute to the varying findings. In a recent study, six capsules containing a total of 1.12 g and 7.56 g of ethyl esters of EPA and DHA respectively, were given daily to 80 patients with stable plaque psoriasis. After eight weeks, approximately 72.4% of the patients completing the study showed moderate to excellent clinical improvement in pruritus, scaling, induration and erythema [16]. An additional study giving a low fat diet supplemented with dietary fish oil (Max-EPA) improved psoriasis accompanied by the formation of LTB_5 [17]. Thus, despite one reported negative result, dietary *n*-3 PUFAs, particularly EPA, seemingly exert minimal to moderate efficacy as a monotherapy for psoriasis. Interestingly, oils or capsules enriched with EPA may prove to be efficatious as an adjunct therapy. For instance, fish oil has been used with success as an adjunct to etretinate therapy in order to reduce the hyperlipidemia caused by etretinate. Furthermore, fish oil capsules have also been used in conjunction with ultraviolet irradiation (UVB) to reduce associated inflammation and to prolong the beneficial effects of phototherapy [18].

Whether *n*-3 PUFAs will become a potent monotherapeutic modality for treatment of psoriasis, and other cutaneous inflammatory/proliferative diseases remains to be determined. To establish true efficacy of *n*-3 PUFAs it is imperative that the mechanisms of action of EPA/DHA as free acids and/or their oxidative metabolites, particularly the monohydroxy fatty acids (15-HEPE and 17-HDoHE) in skin be elucidated. Recent studies using a guinea pig model [5, 19] revealed that the monohydroxy fatty acids generated locally from *n*-3 PUFA fatty acid-monohydroxy fatty acids in the skin, by epidermal 15-lipoxygenase may function as endogenous anti-inflammatory metabolites. These possibilities require further exploration.

A speculative scenario of the possible modulatory effects of EPA/DHA contained in fish oil on the generation of AA inflammatory metabolites via the 5-lipoxygenase pathway of AA metabolism is shown in Figure 3. Pathway [A] illustrates the dietary

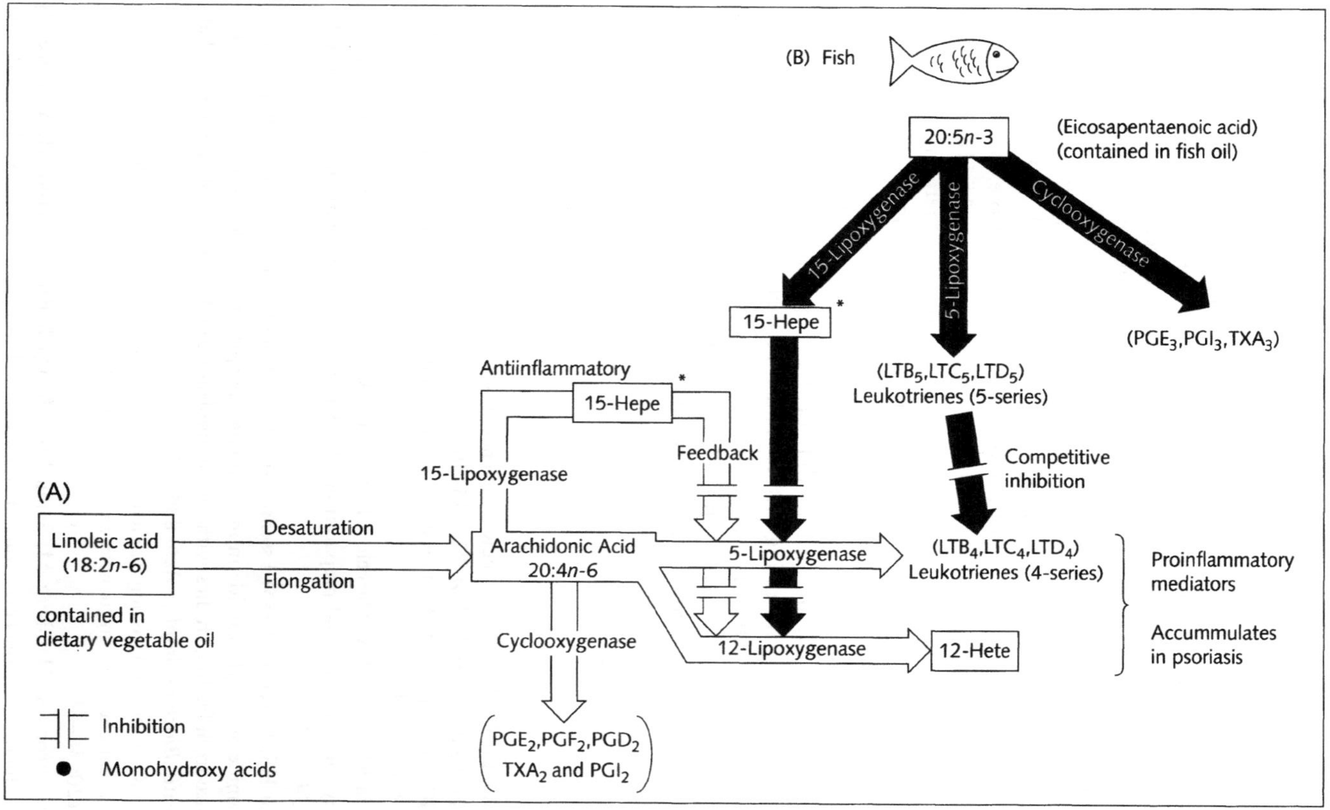

Figure 3
A speculative scenario of the possible modulatory effects of constituent PUFAs in dietary fish oil on the generation of proinflammatory leukotrienes from AA.

ingestion of vegetable oil (safflower or corn oil, containing 18:2*n*-6), its desaturation and elongation into AA. The resulting AA is further metabolized by PMNs via the 5-lipoxygenase into pro-inflammatory leukotrienes, in particular, LTB_4, LTC_4 and LTD_4. Pathway [B] illustrates the oxidative metabolism of fish oil containing EPA/DHA via the cyclooxygenase and lipoxygenase pathways to generate metabolites. The possible mechanisms for the reported beneficial effects of fish oil in some cutaneous disorders seem consistent with the possible *in vivo* epidermal generation of 15-lipoxygenase products of EPA (15-HEPE) and DHA (17-HDoHE). These metabolites have been shown *in vitro* to inhibit the generation of LTB_4 by activated PMNs. The possibility that LTB_5 (a moderate competitor for LTB_4) is formed via the 5-lipoxygenase after dietary intake of fish oil containing EPA also exists, and could attenuate the proinflammatory effects of LTB_4. The increase in 15-HEPE and 17-HDoHE is dose-dependent after dietary intake of fish oil. It is therefore reasonable to speculate that increased dietary ingestion of fish oil (containing EPA/DHA) could result in increased endogenous epidermal biosynthesis of putative anti-inflammatory monohydroxy metabolites, 15-HEPE and 17-HDoHE. Local increase in these monohydroxy acids could in turn inhibit local generation of pro-inflammatory leukotrienes induced by infiltrating PMNs. Thus, the dietary intake of highly purified fish oil or its ethyl esters as a monotherapy or adjunct with other therapeutic modalities may offer a less toxic approach to alleviating cutaneous inflammatory disorders although more studies are still warranted.

References

1 Burr GO, Burr MM (1929) A new deficiency disease produced by the rigid exclusion of fat from the diet. *J Biol Chem* 82: 345–367

2 Burr GO, Burr MM (1930) On the nature of the fatty acids essential in nutrition. *J Biol Chem* 86: 587–621

3 Chapkin RS, Ziboh VA, Marcelo CL, Voorhees JJ (1986) Metabolism of essential fatty acids by human epidermal preparations: Evidence of chain elongation. *J Lipid Res* 27: 945–954

4 Hansen HS, Jensen B (1985) Essential function of linoleic acid esterified in acylglucosylceramide and acylceramide in maintaining the epidermal water permeability barrier. Evidence from feeding studies with oleate, linoleate, arachidonate, columbinate and alinoleneate. *Biochim Biophys Acta* 834: 357–363

5 Miller CC, Ziboh VA, Wong T, Fletcher MP (1990) Dietary supplementation with *n*-3 and *n*-6 enriched oils influences *in vivo* levels of epidermal lipoxygenase products. *J Nutr* 120: 36–44

6 Hammarstrom A, Hamberg M, Samuelsson B, Duell EA, Strawiski M, Voorhees JJ (1975) Increased concentration of nonesterified arachidonic acid. 12L-hydroxy-

5,8,10,14-eicosatetraenoic acid, prostaglandin E_2 and prostaglandin $F_{2\alpha}$ in epidermis of psoriasis. *Proc Natl Acad Sci USA* 72: 5130–5134

7 Brain S, Camp R, Dowd P, Black AK, Greaves M (1984) The release of Leukotriene B_4-like material in biologically active amounts from the lesional skin of patients with psoriasis. *J Invest Dermatol* 83: 70–73

8 Brain S, Camp R, Black AD, Dowd P, Greaves M, Ford-Hutchinson AW (1985) Leukotrienes C_4 and D_4 in psoriatic skin lesions. *Prostaglandins* 29: 611–619

9 Grabbe J, Czarnetzki BM, Rosenbach T, Mardin M (1984) Identification of chemotactic lipoxygenase products of arachidonate metabolism in psoriatic skin. *J Invest Dermatol* 82: 477–479

10 Grabbe J, Rosenbach T, Czarnetzki BM (1985) Production of LTB4-like chemotactic arachidonate metabolites from human keratinocytes. *J Invest Dermatol* 85: 527–530

11 Greaves M, Barr R, Camp R (1984) Leukotriene B_4-like immunoreactivity and skin disease. *Lancet* ii: 160

12 Ziboh VA, Cohen KA, Ellis CN, Miller C, Hamilton TA, Kragballe K, Hydrick CR, Voorhees JJ (1986) Effects of dietary supplementation of fish oil on neutrophil and epidermal fatty acids. *Arch Dermatol* 122: 1277–1282

13 Maurice PDL, Allen BR, Barkley ASJ, Cockbill SR, Stammers J, Bather PC (1987) The effects of dietary supplementation with fish oil in patients with psoriasis. *Br J Dermatol* 117: 599–606

14 Bittiner SB, Cartwright I, Tucker WFG, Bleehen SS (1988) A double-blind randomized placebo-controlled trial of fish oil in psoriasis. *Lancet* 1: 378–380

15 Bjørneboe A, Smith AK, Bjørneboe GE, Thune PO, Drevon CA (1988) Effect of dietary supplementation with *n*-3 fatty acids on clinical manifestations of psoriasis. *Br J Dermatol* 118: 77–83

16 Lassus A, Dahlgren AL, Halpern MJ, Santalahti J, Happonen HP (1990) Effects of dietary supplementation with ethyl ester lipids (angiosan) in patients with psoriasis and psoriatic arthritis. *J International Med Res* 18: 68–73

17 Kragballe K, Fogh K (1989) A low-fat diet supplemented with dietary fish oil (Max-EPA) results in improvement of psoriasis and in formation of leukotriene B_5. *Acta Derm Venereol* 69: 23–28

18 Gupta AK, Ellis CN, Tellner DC, Anderson TF, Voorhees JJ (1989) Double-blind, placebo-controlled study to evaluate the efficacy of fish oil and low-dose UVB in the treatment of psoriasis. *Br J Dermatol* 120: 801–807

19 Miller CC, Ziboh VA (1988) Human epidermis transforms eicosapentaenoic acid to 15-hydroxy-5,8,11,13,17-eicosapentaenoic acid: a potent inhibitor of 5-lipoxygenase activity. *J Am Oil Chem Soc* 65: 474

n-6 Fatty acids and atopic eczema

David F. Horrobin

Scotia Research Institute, Castle Business Park, Stirling, Scotland FK9 4TZ, UK

Introduction

In 1929 and 1930, Burr and Burr reported the development of a scaly dermatitis in rats fed diets free of unsaturated fats [1, 2]. Studies in several animal species and also in humans have now shown that a dietary deficiency of the *n*-6 essential fatty acid (EFA), linoleic acid, but not of the *n*-3 EFA, alpha-linolenic acid, leads to a range of skin abnormalities [3–6]. An inflammatory type of reaction is characteristic, with dryness, then scaling, then a breakdown of the skin surface with redness and weeping. At the same time epidermal cells proliferate more rapidly [7] and the skin becomes highly permeable to water leading to serious water loss across the skin surface [8–10].

In the skin, the EFAs are incorporated into a variety of complex lipids, including ceramides [11, 12] and they can be metabolised to a variety of lipoxygenase and cyclo-oxygenase metabolites [13–17]. In contrast to some other tissues, and notably the liver, the skin cannot convert linoleic acid to arachidonic acid [15, 18, 19]. The first desaturation step of linoleic acid to gamma-linolenic acid (GLA) and the second step of dihomogammalinolenic (DGLA) to arachidonic acid (AA) are both absent. However, the skin can convert GLA to DGLA.

The abnormal skin of *n*-6 EFA deficiency can be demonstrated in humans [3, 20–22]. Hansen, a paediatrician friend of the Burrs, observed that the skin changes in the EFA deficient rats were similar to those in his children who had atopic dermatitis [20–22]. Hansen, in the 1930s, was therefore the first to suggest that atopic dermatitis might be related to abnormal EFA metabolism.

EFA biochemistry in atopic dermatitis

Methods for assaying EFAs in the 1930s were crude, but in his first paper Hansen reported that the iodine number of serum from children with atopic dermatitis was lower than normal, indicating a lower total concentration of EFAs [22]. Later, using

Medicinal Fatty Acids in Inflammation, edited by J.M. Kremer

pooled samples, he concluded that there were reduced levels of both linoleic and arachidonic acids but that only the linoleic acid deficit could be reversed by giving large amounts of dietary linoleic acid [23]. Controversy about the possible reliability and importance of these findings continued in a limited way during the 1930s and 1940s [24, 25] but then stopped for over 30 years, only to be revived with the development of reliable gas chromatography techniques for measuring blood EFAs.

New studies in both adults and children failed to demonstrate any linoleic acid deficiency in blood from atopic eczema patients as compared to normal controls [26, 27]. However, investigators reported that in spite of normal or elevated levels of linoleic acid, there were reduced levels of the linoleic acid metabolites; GLA, DGLA and AA [26–28]. Possible explanations for this include a reduced rate of conversion of linoleic acid to GLA, or alternatively an increased rate of consumption of DGLA and AA, possibly due to inflammatory processes, which cannot be adequately compensated for because of the naturally low rate of conversion of linoleic acid to GLA at the rate-limiting delta-6-desaturation step.

Later, further studies were published in support of this concept. Milk from mothers who had children with atopic eczema had higher than normal levels of linoleic acid and lower than normal levels of metabolites [29]. Similar findings were obtained in adipose tissue of adults with atopic eczema [30] and in red cell membranes [31–32]. Some investigators have not been able to replicate these findings [33, 34]. In Japanese children with eczema there were deficits of linoleic acid, as well as of DGLA and AA [35].

Although there are some conflicts of opinion, most investigators have found reduced levels of linoleic acid metabolites, with less reduction, normality or an elevation of linoleic acid itself. Various investigators have suggested that these abnormalities could lead to reduced formation of prostaglandin Es from DGLA and AA, and hence to the reduced levels of cyclic AMP noted in atopic eczema by other investigators, which could lead to selective hyperactivity in parts of the immune and inflammatory systems [4, 36–39].

Does the skin problem cause or is it caused by the EFA abnormalities?

The reported EFA changes could perhaps be a consequence of widespread inflammatory reactions in the skin consuming DGLA and AA. Alternatively, the EFA changes might actually be responsible for the dermatitis. No definitive answer can yet be given to this question, but one approach might be to see which abnormality can be detected first.

A careful prospective study is relevant to this question [40]. We know that babies are more likely to develop eczema if they have a strong family history. We also know that babies who will later develop eczema have normal skin at birth, with the skin lesions usually appearing only 3–12 months later. Galli et al. [40] therefore took blood samples from the umbilical cord and at one and three months, from 57 babies born to mothers where there was an eczema family history. The infants were then monitored for the remainder of the year and at 12 months it was decided whether or not the child had atopic eczema. This was then related to the EFA blood levels at birth, one month and three months.

Almost half the babies developed atopic eczema. When the babies who did and who did not have eczema were compared, the differences in EFA levels at birth were clear cut. The babies who later developed eczema had significantly elevated linoleic acid levels and significantly low levels of DGLA and AA. Thus, in this group, the EFA abnormalities clearly preceded the development of the skin condition [40].

Such an EFA abnormality could lead to skin lesions by two routes. First, there may be direct effects on the skin because of the reduced levels of DGLA and AA. Second, there may be a sensitisation of the immune system leading to skin damage by immunological mechanisms. The first might be easily reversible by treatment with the missing EFAs. The second might be irreversible or difficult to reverse by EFA treatment.

Treatment with linoleic acid

The pathways of linoleic acid metabolism through to DGLA and AA were not worked out in the 1930s and 1940s, nor was the distinction between the *n*-6 and *n*-3 EFAs understood. Most unsaturated fatty acids were thought to have similar actions. The unsaturated fatty acid sources available to Hansen and his colleagues were what we now know to be sources of linoleic acid, for example, lard and vegetable oils, or cod liver oil which is largely a source of *n*-3 EFAs.

After Hansen's work there were many therapeutic trials of unsaturated fatty acids in atopic eczema. Those investigators who happened to use cod liver oil had poor results [42–44]. Those who used sources of linoleic acid obtained good results but only with astronomical doses of 10-60 g of linoleic acid per day [25, 45–47]. These doses were far higher than those needed to reverse the skin lesions of EFA deficiency. Lower doses were ineffective [48].

With hindsight we can understand these observations. *n*-3 EFAs are now known to be of little importance in the skin compared to *n*-6 EFAs, and so it is not surprising that cod liver oil failed. The modern studies have, for the most part, shown that any deficit is not in linoleic acid but in linoleic acid metabolites. It is therefore not surprising that linoleic acid does not work at low doses, especially since Hansen showed that linoleic acid treatment did not change AA concentrations [25]. The astronomical doses of linoleic acid which were effective may have been needed to force formation of enough metabolites beyond the rate-limiting delta-6-desaturase step. If this explanation is correct, then by-passing that step with GLA should be more effective.

GLA treatment: Biochemical and objective effects

GLA has now been administered to patients in a number of studies in the form of a specific variety of evening primrose oil (Epogam). This, unlike other vegetable oils which usually contain linoleic acid as their only *n*-6 EFA, contains 9% GLA. Administration of 2 g, 4 g or 6 g/day of evening primrose oil (EPO) produced a significant dose-related rise in plasma-phospholipid DGLA in adult patients with atopic eczema, together with a less consistent rise in AA [26]. In Japanese children with atopic eczema, GLA administration normalised the blood EFA profile [35]. In adults, 2 g, 4 g, and 6 g of EPO/day produced dose-related increase in DGLA and AA both in skin phospholipids and in blood neutrophils [49]. Thus the abnormal blood and tissue fatty acid levels in atopic eczema can be partially corrected by relatively low doses of GLA. The changes in DGLA levels have consistently been greater than the changes in AA, probably because of the rate-limiting nature of delta-5-desaturation.

The mechanisms of any putative anti-inflammatory effects remain a matter for speculation but there are several possibilities. DGLA can be converted to prostaglandin E_1 which can elevate cyclic AMP and inhibit phospholipase [36–39]. DGLA can also be metabolised to 15-OH-DGLA which is an inhibitor of lipoxygenases and hence of leukotriene formation [11, 50–52]. An entirely different mechanism may relate to suppression of interleukin-2 receptor levels which has been noted following EPO treatment in eczema patients [53].

Other abnormalities in atopic eczema patients which can be objectively assessed include elevated blood catecholamine levels, and the roughness of the apparently normal skin areas such as the inside of the forearm. EPO, but not control treatment, significantly reduced the elevated noradrenaline and adrenaline levels in patients with atopic eczema [54]. Two studies have been performed to investigate by objective profilometry techniques the effects of EPO on skin roughness. In both studies there was a significant reduction in the roughness of the skin, bringing it within the normal range [56, 57].

Clinical results of gamma-linolenic acid treatment

A pilot study of GLA treatment for three weeks showed a modest beneficial effect [58]. This was followed by a randomised, placebo-controlled study of Epogam at three daily dose levels in adults (2 g, 4 g and 6 g) and two in children (1 g and 2 g). In this second study, active treatment produced significant and dose-related beneficial effects [59]. A further randomised study showed both a beneficial clinical effect and a significant reduction in topical steroid use in the EPO group [60]. The placebo-treated patients required three times more steroid to control their condition than did the EPO patients.

EPO seems to be particularly beneficial in very young children. Strong therapeutic effects were reported in a placebo-controlled study and it was shown that these results were sustained in long term use [61–63]. Positive therapeutic effects using EPO in placebo-controlled studies were also reported with topical EPO [64] and, with oral EPO in hyperactivity associated with eczema [65], in adults with atopic dermatitis [66] and in women with pre-menstrual exacerbations of eczema [67]. Two substantial negative studies have also been reported [68, 69]. However, in the second of these, the results using a validated standard scoring system were inexplicably omitted. On including these omitted results, a significant beneficial effect of EPO was demonstrable: moreover, on stopping treatment the improvements noted in the placebo group were rapidly reversed, whereas those in the EPO group persisted for four weeks after the trial, leading to a clearly significant difference between the groups at this point [70–72]. A meta-analysis showed a highly significant difference between active and placebo groups, particularly with regard to the symptom of itch [73]. Itch is an exceptionally important feature of atopic eczema. It is the most distressing aspect of the condition from the patientís view point, and the consequent scratching promotes the skin inflammation. EPO is the only treatment which has been shown to reduce itch significantly.

Most patients with eczema are treated with topical steroids. Ethical committees have usually refused to allow steroid treatment to be stopped in order to allow a straight comparison between GLA and placebo. Thus most of the studies have in fact been directed to testing whether or not GLA or placebo has significant benefits over and above the effects of topical steroids. This is a severe trial, especially since steroids may interfere with the effects of GLA by blocking the mobilisation of GLA and DGLA from membrane phospholipids. When all the 22 studies of GLA, published and unpublished, are ranked in relation to the background use of steroids, some interesting trends are observed. Table 1 shows this when the studies are divid-

Table 1 - Effects of treatment with GLA in twenty two randomised, placebo-controlled trials divided according to whether patients were receiving as background treatment emollients and hydrocortisone only, or steroids more potent than hydrocortisone

	Percentage of studies with patients using	
Study outcome	**More potent steroids**	**Emollients/hydrocortisone**
No effect	33% (3)	0% (0)
Trend in favour of GLA	44% (4)	38% (5)
Significant beneficial effect of GLA	22% (2)	62% (8)

ed into those where the background medication was either an emollient or a mild steroid (hydrocortisone) or when the background medication was a more potent steroid. When more potent steroids were used, 66% of the studies showed a beneficial effect but in only 22% was this significant. When only mild steroids or emollients were used, all studies showed a beneficial effects and in 62% this was significant. Thus GLA is considerably more effective in the absence of steroids or when only the lowest potency steroids are used.

Conclusions

There is reasonable evidence that there are biochemical abnormalities in *n*-6 EFA metabolism in atopic eczema and that these abnormalities precede the onset of the illness. These abnormalities can be partially corrected by the administration of GLA as evening primrose oil. GLA produces improvements in skin smoothness and in blood catecholamine levels and also has a modest clinical therapeutic effect especially in the absence of co-treatment with potent steroids.

References

1 Burr GO, Burr MM (1929) A new deficiency disease produced by the rigid exclusion of fat from the diet. *J Biol Chem* 82: 345–367

2 Burr GO, Burr MM (1930) On the nature and role of the fatty acids essential in nutrition. *J Biol Chem* 86: 587–621

3 Sheretz EF (1986) The Skin and Essential Fatty Acid Deficiency. In: DA Roe (ed): *Nutrition and the Skin.* Alan R. Liss, New York, 117–130

4 Horrobin DF (1989) Essential fatty acids in clinical dermatology. *J Am Acad Dermatol* 20: 1045–1053

5 Wright S (1991) Essential fatty acids and the skin. *Br J Dermatol* 125: 503–515

6 Burton JL (1989) Dietary fatty acids and inflammatory skin disease. *Lancet* 1: 27–31

7 Lowe NJ, DeQuoy PR (1978) Linoleic acid effects on epidermal DNA synthesis and cutaneous prostaglandin levels in essential fatty acid deficiency. *J Invest Dermatol* 70: 200–203

8 Basnayake V, Sinclair HM (1954) Skin permeability in deficiency of essential fatty acids. *J Physiol* 126: 55P–56P

9 Hartop PJ, Prottey C (1976) Changes in transepidermal water loss and the composition of epidermal lecithin after applications of pure fatty acid triglycerides to skin of essential fatty acid-deficient rats. *Br J Dermatol* 95: 255–264

10 Prottey C (1977) Investigation of functions of essential fatty acids in the skin. *Br J Dermatol* 97: 29–38

11 Ziboh VA (1987) Biochemical abnormalities in essential fatty acid deficiency. *Models Dermatol* 3: 106–111
12 Bowser PA, Nugteren DH, White RJ, Houtsmuller UM, Prottey C (1985) Identification, isolation and characterization of epidermal lipids containing linoleic acid. *Biochim Biophys Acta* 834: 419–428
13 Ziboh VA, Chapkin RS (1987) Biologic significance of polyunsaturated fatty acids in the skin. *Arch Dermatol* 123: 1686a–1690a
14 Ziboh VA (1994) Essential fatty acids/eicosanoid biosynthesis in the skin: biological significance. *Proc Soc Exp Biol Med* 205: 1–11
15 Ziboh VA, Miller CC (1990) Essential fatty acids and polyunsaturated fatty acids: significance in cutaneous biology. *Annu Rev Nutr* 10: 433–450
16 Nugteren DH, Christ Hazelhof E, van der Beek A, Houtsmuller UM (1985) Metabolism of linoleic acid and other essential fatty acids in the epidermis of the rat. *Biochim Biophys Acta* 834: 429–436
17 Kassis V (1983) The prostaglandin system in human skin. *Dan Med Bull* 30: 320–343
18 Chapkin RS, Ziboh VA (1984) Inability of skin enzyme preparations to biosynthesize arachidonic acid from linoleic acid. *Biochem Biophys Res Commun* 124: 784–792
19 Chapkin RS, Ziboh VA, Marcelo CL, Voorhees JJ (1986) Metabolism of essential fatty acids by human epidermal enzyme preparations: evidence of chain elongation. *J Lipid Res* 27: 945–954
20 Hansen AE, Haggard ME, Boelesche AN, Adam D, Wiese HF (1958) Essential fatty acids in infant nutrition III. Clinical manifestations of linoleic acid deficiency. *J Nutr* 66: 565–576
21 Hansen AE, Wiese HF (1954) Essential fatty acids and human nutrition II. Serum level for unsaturated fatty acids in poorly nourished infants and children. *J Nutr* 52: 367–374
22 Hansen AE (1933) Study of iodine number of serum fatty acids in infantile eczema. *Proc Soc Exper Biol Med* 30: 1198–1199
23 Brown WR, Hansen AE (1937) Arachidonic acid and linoleic acid of the serum in normal and eczematous human subjects. *Proc Soc Exp Biol Med* 30: 113–116
24 Faber HK, Roberts DB (1933) Studies in infantile allergic eczema II. Serum lipids, with special reference to saturation of the fatty acids. *J Pediatr* 3: 490–493
25 Hansen AE, Knott EM, Wiese HF, Shaperman E, McQuarrie I (1947) Eczema and essential fatty acids. *Am J Dis Child* 73: 1–18
26 Manku MS, Horrobin DF, Morse N, Kyte V, Jenkins K (1982) Reduced levels of prostaglandin precursors in the blood of atopic patients: defective delta-6-desaturase function as a biochemical basis for atopy. *Prostaglandins Leukot Med* 9: 615–628
27 Manku MS, Horrobin DF, Morse NL, Wright S, Burton JL (1984) Essential fatty acids in the plasma phospholipids of patients with atopic eczema. *Br J Dermatol* 110: 643–648
28 Strannegard IL, Svennerholm L, Strannegard O (1987) Essential fatty acids in serum lecithin of children with atopic dermatitis and in umbilical cord serum of infants with high or low IgE levels. *Int Arch Allergy Appl Immunol* 82: 422–423

29 Wright S, Bolton C (1989) Breast milk fatty acids in mothers of children with atopic eczema. *Br J Nutr* 62: 693–697
30 Wright S, Sanders TA (1991) Adipose tissue essential fatty acid composition in patients with atopic eczema. *Eur J Clin Nutr* 45: 501–505
31 Oliwiecki S, Burton JL, Elles K, Horrobin DF (1991) Levels of essential and other fatty acids in plasma and red cell phospholipids from normal controls and patients with atopic eczema. *Acta Derm Venereol* 71: 224–228
32 Biagi PL, Hrelia S, Celadon M, Bordoni A (1993) Erythrocyte membrane fatty acid composition in children with atopic dermatitis compared to age-matched controls. *Acta Paediatr* 82: 789–790
33 Yu G, Kjellman N-I, Bjorksten B (1996) Phospholipid fatty acids in cord blood: family history and development of allergy. *Acta Paediatr* 85: 679–683
34 Sakai K, Ueno K, Ogawa Y, Okuyama H (1986) Fatty acid compositions of plasma lipids in young atopic patients. *Chem Pharm Bull* 34: 2944–2949
35 Shimasaki H (1995) PUFA content and effect of dietary intake of gamma-linolenic acid-rich oil on profiles of *n*-6, *n*-3 metabolites in plasma of children with atopic eczema. *J Clin Biochem Nutr* 19: 183–192
36 Wright S (1985) Atopic dermatitis and essential fatty acids: a biochemical basis for atopy? *Acta Derm Venereol* 114 (Suppl): 143–145
37 Wright S (1991) Essential fatty acids and atopic dermatitis. *Pediatr Allergy Immunol* 2 (Suppl 1): 23–30
38 Melnik BC, Plewig G (1990) Atopy: a prostaglandin E precursor- and receptor-dependent defect in T-cell maturation and function? *Br J Dermatol* 123: 126–128
39 Melnik BC, Plewig G (1989) Is the origin of atopy linked to deficient conversion of omega-6-fatty acids to prostaglandin E1? *J Am Acad Dermatol* 21: 557–563
40 Galli E, Picardo M, Chini L et al (1994) Analysis of polyunsaturated fatty acids in newborn sera: a screening tool for atopic disease? *Br J Dermatol* 130: 752–756
41 Hansen AE (1937) Serum lipids in eczema and other pathological conditions. *Amer J Dis Child* 53: 933–946
42 Taub SJ, Zakon SJ (1935) The use of unsaturated fatty acids in the treatment of eczema. *J Am Med Assoc* 105: 1675
43 Epstein NN, Glick D (1937) Unsaturated fatty acids in eczema. Observations on acne vulgaris, psoriasis, xanthoma tuberosum and xanthoma palpebrarum. *Arch Dermatol Syph* 35: 427–432
44 Ginsberg JE, Bernstein C, Iob LV (1937) Effects of oils containing unsaturated fatty acids on patients with dermatitis. *Arch Dermatol Syph* 36: 1033–1038
45 Hansen AE, Wiese HF, Boelsche AN, Haggard ME, Adam DJD, Davis H (1963) Role of linoleic acid in infant nutrition. Clinical and chemical study of 428 infants fed on milk mixtures varying in kinds and amount fat. *Pediatrics* 31: 171–192
46 Cornbleet T (1935) Use of maize oil (unsaturated fatty acids) in the treatment of eczema. *Arch Dermatol Syph* 31: 224–226

47 Finnerud CW, Kesler RL, Wiese HF (1941) Ingestion of lard in the treatment of eczema and allied dermatoses. *Arch Dermatol Syph* 44: 849–861

48 Pettit JHS (1954) Use of unsaturated fatty acids in the eczemas of childhood. *Br Med J* 1: 79–81

49 Schafer L, Kragballe K (1991) Supplementation with evening primrose oil in atopic dermatitis: effect on fatty acids in neutrophils and epidermis. *Lipids* 26: 557–560

50 Ziboh VA (1992) Prostaglandins, leukotrienes, and hydroxy fatty acids in epidermis. *Semin Dermatol* 11: 114–120

51 Ziboh VA (1996) The significance of polyunsaturated fatty acids in cutaneous biology. *Lipids* 31: 249–253

52 Chapkin RS, Ziboh VA, McCullough JL (1987) Dietary influences of evening primrose and fish oil on the skin of essential fatty acid-deficient guinea pigs. *J Nutr* 117: 1360–1370

53 Ziboh VA (1989) Implications of dietary oils and polyunsaturated fatty acids in the management of cutaneous disorders. *Arch Dermatol* 125: 241–245

54 Humphreys F, Symonds JA, Duff GW, Hunter JAA (1997) *The effects of evening primrose oil on SIL2 receptor levels in atopic eczema.* British Association of Dermatology Annual Meeting

55 Courage B, Nissen HP, Wehrmann W, Biltz H (1991) Influence of polyunsaturated fatty acids on the plasma catecholamines of patients with atopic eczema. *Z Hautkr* 66: 509–510

56 Nissen HP, Wehrmann W, Kroll U, Kreysel HW (1988) Influence of polyunsaturated fatty acids on the plasma phospholipids of atopic patients. *Fat Sci Technol* 90: 268–271

57 Marshall RJ, Evans RW (1990) Measurement of the effects of essential fatty acids on human skin smoothness. In: DF Horrobin (ed): *Omega-6 Essential Fatty Acids: Pathophysiology and Roles in Clinical Medicine.* Alan R. Liss, New York, 81–98

58 Lovell CR, Burton JL, Horrobin DF (1981) Treatment of atopic eczema with evening primrose oil. *Lancet* 1: 278

59 Wright S, Burton JL (1982) Oral evening-primrose-seed oil improves atopic eczema. *Lancet* 2: 1120–1122

60 Schalin-Karrila M, Mattila L, Jansen CT, Uotila P (1987) Evening primrose oil in the treatment of atopic eczema: effect on clinical status, plasma phospholipid fatty acids and circulating blood prostaglandins. *Br J Dermatol* 117: 11–19

61 Bordoni A, Biagi PL, Masi M, Ricci G, Fanelli C, Patrizi A, Ceccolini E (1988) Evening primrose oil (Efamol) in the treatment of children with atopic eczema. *Drugs Exp Clin Res* 14: 291–297

62 Biagi PL, Bordoni A, Masi M, Ricci G, Fanelli C, Patrizi A, Ceccolini E (1988) A long-term study on the use of evening primrose oil (Efamol) in atopic children. *Drugs Exp Clin Res* 14: 285–290

63 Biagi PL, Bordoni A, Hrelia S et al (1994) The effect of gamma-linolenic acid on clinical status, red cell fatty acid composition and membrane microviscosity in infants with atopic dermatitis. *Drugs Exp Clin Res* 20: 77–84

64 Anstey A, Quigley M, Wilkinson JD (1991) Topical evening primrose oil as treatment for atopic eczema. *J Dermatol Treatment* 1: 199–201

65 Guenther L, Wexler D (1987) Efamol in the treatment of atopic dermatitis. *J Am Acad Dermatol* 17: 860

66 Meigel W (1985) Treatment of atopic dermatitis. *Z Hautkr* 61: 473–478

67 Humphreys F, Symons JA, Brown HK, Duff GN, Hunter JA (1994) The effects of gamolenic acid on adult atopic eczema and premenstrual exacerbation of eczema. *Eur J Dermatol* 4: 598–603

68 Bamford JTM, Gibson RW, Renier CM (1985) Atopic eczema unresponsive to evening primrose oil (linoleic and gamma-linolenic acids). *J Am Acad Dermatol* 13: 959–965

69 Berth-Jones J, Graham-Brown RAC (1993) Placebo-controlled trial of essential fatty acid supplementation in atopic dermatitis. *Lancet* 341: 1557–1560

70 Horrobin DF, Stewart C (1990) Evening primrose oil in atopic eczema. *Lancet* 335: 864–865

71 Horrobin DF, Stewart C (1990) Evening primrose oil and atopic eczema. *Lancet* 336: 50

72 Horrobin DF, Morse PF (1995) Evening primrose oil and atopic eczema. *Lancet* 345: 260–261

73 Morse PF, Horrobin DF, Manku MS et al (1989) Meta-analysis of placebo-controlled studies of the efficacy of Epogam in the treatment of atopic eczema. Relationship between plasma essential fatty acid changes and clinical response. *Br J Dermatol* 121: 75–90

n-6 Fatty acids and nervous system disorders

David F. Horrobin

Scotia Research Institute, Castle Business Park, Stirling, Scotland FK9 4TZ, UK

Introduction

The relationship between n-6 essential fatty acids (EFAs) and nervous system disorders is a subject of emerging interest. In one specific area, the peripheral neuropathy of diabetes, the role of n-6 EFAs is now well established. In other areas, including schizophrenia and dyskinesias, much less work has been done although there is tantalising evidence that n-6 EFAs may be involved. This review will primarily concentrate on diabetic neuropathy with a short section drawing attention to the few key papers in these disorders.

Peifer and Holman [1] reported that diabetic animals required a much higher than normal amount of dietary linoleic acid to counteract the signs of EFA deficiency. Brenner et al. [2] provided a possible explanation when they reported that in diabetic animals the conversion of linoleic acid to gamma-linolenic acid (GLA) was markedly impaired, leading to reduced supply of the further metabolites, dihomogamma-linolenic acid (DGLA) and arachidonic acid (AA). In animal models this deficit has been repeatedly confirmed (reviewed in [3–5]). There is no direct evidence of impaired delta-6-desaturation in humans but considerable indirect evidence. In type I diabetes in particular, the amount of blood EFA is similar to that in diabetic animals, with elevated levels of linoleic acid and reduced levels of linoleic acid metabolites, including DGLA and AA (reviewed in [4–6]).

Neuropathy is one of the commonest complications of both type I and type II diabetes. In particular it leads to loss of peripheral sensori-motor function. The absence of cutaneous sensation leads to impaired skin circulation and loss of the ability to detect minor mechanical and thermal trauma. This in turn leads to skin ulcers which are difficult to heal, and frequently this leads to eventually to ulceration and gangrene.

Although many different mechanisms have been proposed for the nerve damage, one involving the role of EFAs in neuronal structure and function and in nerve microcirculation is currently gaining importance [5–8]. DGLA and AA are required for the normal structure of neuronal membranes, and without such normal struc-

Medicinal Fatty Acids in Inflammation, edited by J.M. Kremer

ture, normal function is impossible. The EFAs are required for nerve conduction, partly via their involvement in the phosphatidyl-inositol/calcium cycle, and partly because of the importance of DGLA and AA-derived prostaglandins in nerve conduction [8]. With regard to the nerve microcirculation, prostaglandin E_1 from DGLA and prostacyclin from AA both play important roles as vasodilators. For these and other reasons, impaired conversion of linoleic acid to GLA could play a major long term role in contributing to nerve damage in diabetes. If so, by-passing the impaired metabolic step described by Brenner et al. by providing GLA directly may have beneficial effects.

Animal studies of GLA

The rat with streptozotocin-induced diabetes is widely used as a model for human type I diabetes. These rats develop diabetic neuropathy which in some respects is similar to that in humans. However, the rat model is much more acute and may not reflect well the long term types of change seen in humans with both types of diabetes. With these reservations, the rat may be used as a guide to the human condition.

Investigators have studied the effects of GLA on rat diabetic neuropathy. The results are very consistent and all investigators have demonstrated clear beneficial effects. GLA is able both to prevent and to reverse the nerve damage [9–16].

Much attention has been paid to impaired nerve blood flow which seems to be one of the key mechanisms producing neuronal damage in animals. The reduced blood flow is associated with reduced formation of prostacyclin from AA and also with reduced production of nitric oxide. It is therefore of great interest that the impaired nerve conduction, reduced nerve blood flow, and reduced nerve prostacyclin and nitric oxide levels can all be simultaneously corrected by the provision of GLA [11–17]. This suggests that Brenner's idea, that impaired delta-6-desaturation plays a fundamental role in the development of diabetic complications, may be correct, at least as far as neuropathy is concerned.

The initial studies were all carried out on evening primrose oil (EPO) which contains 9% GLA, much of it in the form of a triglyceride, dilinoleoyl-mono-γ-linolenyl-glycerol (DLMG) containing two molecules of linoleic acid and one of GLA [18). Dines et al. tested whether the effects of EPO could be explained by GLA, by purifying DLMG from evening primrose oil and also by making a pure tri-GLA triglyceride. They then performed careful dose response studies of EPO, DLMG and tri-GLA [19]. When plotted in terms of GLA content, the three curves could be directly superimposed, indicating that the EPO effect really was attributable to GLA.

However, not all GLA-containing oils behave similarly. Borage oil (22% GLA), blackcurrant oil (16% GLA) and fungal oil (19% GLA) were all tested in the same system [20, 21]. The GLA in these oils was much less effective than either EPO, or pure GLA or DLMG. This indicates one of the pitfalls of using natural oils as sources of particular fatty acids. Presumably some other component of the oil is interfering with the effect of the GLA, so leading to unexpected results [22–24]. This sort of problem may well contribute to the highly variable clinical and biological effects which have been reported for both *n*-6 and *n*-3 EFA-containing oils. In only a few of these studies have standardised oils been used. Full evaluation of the true biomedical effects of EFAs will require the availability of standardised EFA preparations.

Human biochemical studies

There is good evidence that, in type I diabetes, the defects in EFA metabolism are similar to those seen in rats with diabetes. Although there are no direct studies of EFA desaturation in humans with diabetes, there are studies which show that linoleic acid levels in blood are normal or elevated, whereas the levels of the metabolites GLA, DGLA and AA are substantially reduced [4–6, 25–27].

There has until recently been no equivalent evidence for type II diabetes. However, a large study has now compared both plasma and red cell fatty acid profiles in 319 normal controls, 224 type I diabetic patients and 364 type II diabetic patients [28]. In type I patients, in both plasma and red cells there was a marked elevation of the ratio of the concentrations of linoleic acid to those of its metabolites, GLA, DGLA and AA. This is consistent with Brenner's proposal. In type II diabetes, the changes were similar but quantitatively very much less marked, providing less evidence of impaired desaturation. What was particularly striking was that in both groups the red cell concentrations of DGLA and AA were reduced to a very much greater extent than the plasma concentrations.

This suggests that in both types of diabetes, superimposed on any problems with desaturation, there is a marked impairment of the transfer of highly unsaturated EFAs from plasma into cell membranes [28].

Human studies of diabetic neuropathy

Three randomised, placebo-controlled trials with the administration of GLA as EPO to humans with diabetic neuropathy have now been performed. In each study 480 mg of GLA or placebo was provided each day in soft gelatin capsules. The first pilot study was conducted over six months and strongly suggested a beneficial effect of GLA [29]. As a result, two large multicentre trials of near-identical design were set up. In each case, patients with established mild to moderate diabetic neuropathy were randomised to receive GLA or placebo for a period of 12 months. Six neurophysiological parameters (motor nerve conduction velocity, sensory nerve conduction velocity, motor nerve action potential amplitude, sensory nerve action potential amplitude, F wave latency and compound muscle action potential), hot and cold quantitative thermal thresholds, and six clinical parameters (light touch, pain, joint sense, vibration sense, reflexes, muscle strength) were measured in upper and lower limbs, making twenty eight parameters in all.

The results in the two trials were very similar. In the first trial involving 111 patients in 7 centres, 26 of 28 parameters were better with GLA than with placebo [30]. In the second trial, involving 293 patients in 10 centres, 27 of 28 parameters showed a better response to active treatment [31]. When both trials were combined, all 28 parameters were better on active treatment, 25 significantly so [31].

These two trials are consistent with the animal work and with Brenner's original hypothesis that impaired *n*-6 EFA metabolism may be important in diabetic complications.

Other nervous system abnormalities

The evidence in other areas is tentative and much less complete. However, each case indicates that further work is required.

In schizophrenia there is evidence that there is accelerated loss of EFAs from membrane phospholipids, leading to decreased levels of both *n*-6 and *n*-3 EFAs in cell membranes. This loss could have a number of causes including increased phospholipase activities [32] or increased oxidation due to impaired antioxidant defence systems [33]. Direct evidence of a functional deficit of AA has recently been obtained by studying the effect of topical application of niacin on cutaneous flushing. In normal individuals, in less than a minute this produces a dose-related increase in skin circulation due to release of membrane AA and its conversion to the vasodilator, prostaglandin D_2 [34]. In approximately 70% of individuals with schizophrenia this response is markedly impaired, indicating a reduced availability of AA [34].

Dyskinesias are abnormal involuntary movements which have been thought to be related primarily to psychotropic drug use. However, careful general population studies have shown that mild to moderate dyskinesias are in fact quite common as people age, even in the absence of drug use. A recent large study involving 446 sixty year old men, showed that smoking and, especially, low plasma phospholipid AA levels were significant predictors of dyskinesia risk [35]. The association with low blood AA was very highly significant ($p < 0.0001$).

Conclusions

Both *n*-6 and *n*-3 EFAs are major components of both central and peripheral nervous systems. They both have important structural and functional roles. It would not be surprising if abnormal EFA metabolism played a role in several nervous system disorders. The evidence is particularly strong in the case of diabetic neuropathy. However, the early evidence in relation to schizophrenia and dyskinesias suggests promising lines of investigation.

References

1 Peifer JJ, Holman RT (1955) Essential fatty acids, diabetes and cholesterol. *Arch Biochem Biophys* 57: 520–521

2 Mercuri O, Peluffo RO, Brenner RR (1966) Depression of microsomal desaturation of linoleic to gamma-linolenic acid in the alloxan diabetic rat. *Biochim Biophys Acta* 116: 407–411

3 Brenner RR (1982) Nutritional and hormonal factors influencing desaturation of essential fatty acids. *Progr Lipid Res* 20: 41–48

4 Horrobin DF (1992) Nutritional and medical importance of gamma-linolenic acid. *Progr Lipid Res* 31: 163-194

5 Horrobin DF (1988) The roles of essential fatty acids in the development of diabetic neuropathy and other complications of diabetes mellitus. *Prostaglandins, Leukotr Essential Fatty Acids* 31: 181–197

6 Horrobin DF (ed) (1992) *Treatment of Diabetic Neuropathy: A New Approach.* Churchill Livingstone, Edinburgh and New York

7 Jamal GA (1994) The use of gamma linolenic acid in the prevention and treatment of diabetic neuropathy. *Diabetic Med* 11: 145–149

8 Horrobin DF, Durand LG, Manku MS (1977) Prostaglandin E_1 modifies nerve conduction and interferes with local anaesthetic action. *Prostaglandins* 14: 103–110

9 Julu POO (1988) Essential fatty acids prevent slowed nerve conduction velocity in streptozotocin diabetes rats. *J Diabetic Comp* 2: 185–188

10 Julu POO (1992) Responses of peripheral nerve conduction velocities to treatment with essential fatty acids in diabetic rats: possible mechanisms of action. In: DF Horrobin (ed): *Treatment of diabetic neuropathy: a new approach.* Churchill Livingstone, Edinburgh and New York, 41–62

11 Tomlinson DR, Robinson JP, Compton AM, Keen P (1989) Essential fatty acid treatment – effects on nerve conduction, polyol pathway and axonal transport in streptozotocin diabetic rats. *Diabetologia* 32: 655–659

12 Stevens EJ, Lockett MJ, Carrington AL, Tomlinson DR (1993) Essential fatty acids treatment prevents nerve ischaemia and associated conduction anomalies in rats with experimental diabetes mellitus. *Diabetologia* 36: 397–401

13 Stevens EJ, Carrington AL, Tomlinson DR (1993) Prostacyclin release in experimental diabetes: effects of evening primrose oil. *Prostaglandins Leukotr Essential Fatty Acids* 49: 699–706

14 Cameron NE, Cotter MA, Robertson S (1991) Essential fatty acid diet supplementation.

Effects on peripheral nerve and skeletal muscle function and capillarization in streptozocin-induced diabetic rats. *Diabetes* 40: 532–539

15 Dines KC, Cotter MA, Cameron NE (1993) Contrasting effects of treatment with ω-3 and ω-6 essential fatty acids on peripheral nerve function and capillarization in streptozotocin-diabetic rats. *Diabetologia* 36: 1132–1138

16 Cameron NE, Cotter MA (1993) Potential therapeutic approaches to the treatment or prevention of diabetic neuropathy: evidence from experimental studies. *Diabetic Med* 10: 593–605

17 Omawari N, Mahmood S, Dewhurst M, Stevens EJ, Tomlinson DR (1995) Deficient nitric oxide is responsible for reduced nerve blood flow in diabetic rats: prevention by essential fatty acids. *Br J Pharmacol* 116: 63

18 Redden PR, Lin XR, Fahey J, Horrobin DF (1995) Stereospecific analysis of the major triacylglycerol species containing gamma-linolenic acid in evening primrose oil and borage oil. *J Chromatography* 704: 99–111

19 Dines KC, Cameron NE, Cotter MA (1995) Comparison of the effects of evening primrose oil and triglycerides containing γ-linolenic acid on nerve conduction and blood flow in diabetic rats. *J Pharmacol Exp Ther* 273: 49–55

20 Dines KC Cotter MA, Cameron NE (1996) Effectiveness of natural oils as sources of gamma-linolenic acid to correct peripheral nerve conduction velocity abnormalities in diabetic rats: modulation by thromboxane A2 inhibition. *Prostaglandins Leukotr Essent Fatty Acids* 55: 159–165

21 Dines KC (1994) *Effects of oils containing gamma-linolenic acid on nerve function in diabetic rats*. PhD Thesis, University of Aberdeen

22 Jenkins DK, Mitchell JC, Manku MS, Horrobin, DF (1988) Effects of different sources of gamma-linolenic acid on the formation of essential fatty acid and prostanoid metabolites. *Med Sci Res* 16: 525–526

23 Fan Y-Y, Chapkin RS (1992) Mouse peritoneal macrophage prostaglandin E_1 synthesis is altered by dietary gamma-linolenic acid. *J Nutr* 122: 1600–1606

24 Horrobin DF (1994) Natural does not equal safe. *Pharmaceutical Tech Europe,* December 14–15

25 Van Doormaal JJ, Idema IG, Muskiet FAJ, Martini IA, Doorenbos H (1988) Effects of short-term high dose intake of evening primrose oil on plasma and cellular fatty acid compositions, a-tocopherol levels, and erythropoiesis in normal and Type I (insulin-dependent) diabetic men. *Diabetologia* 31: 576–584

26 Tilvis RS, Miettinen TA (1985) Fatty acid composition of serum lipids erythrocytes and platelets in insulin-dependent diabetic women. *J Clin Endocr Metabol* 61: 741–745

27 Arisaka M, Arisaka O, Fukuda Y, Yamashiro Y (1986) Prostaglandin metabolism in children with diabetes mellitus. I. Plasma prostaglandin E_2, F_2a, TxB_2 and serum fatty acid levels. *J Paed Gastroenterol Nutr* 5: 878–882

28 Horrobin DF (1997) Essential fatty acid metabolism in patients with diabetic neuropathy. *Prostaglandins Leukotr EFAs* 57: 256

29 Jamal GA, Carmichael H (1990) The effect of γ linolenic acid on human diabetic peripheral neuropathy: a double-blind placebo-controlled trial. *Diabetic Med* 7: 319– 323
30 The Gamma-linolenic Acid Multicenter Trial Group (1993) Treatment of diabetic neuropathy with γ-linolenic acid. *Diabetes Care* 16: 8–15
31 Gamma-linolenic Acid Multicenter Trial Group (Boulton AJ) (1997) Two multicentre double blind trials of gamolenic acid in diabetic peripheral sensori motor neuropathy. *Prostaglandins Leukotr EFAs* 57: 201
32 Horrobin DF Glen AI, Vaddadi K (1994) The membrane hypothesis of schizophrenia. *Schizophr Res* 13: 195–207
33 Mahhadik SP, Gowda S (1996) Antioxidants in the treatment of schizophrenia. *Drugs Today* 32: 553–565
34 Ward P, Sutherland J, Glen E, Glen I (1998) Niacin skin flush in schizophrenia. *Schizophr Res* 29: 269–274
35 Nilsson A, Horrobin DF, Rosengren A, Waller L, Adlerberth A, Wilhelmsen L (1996) Essential fatty acids and abnormal involuntary movements in the general male population: a study of men born in 1933. *Prostaglandins Leukotr EFAs* 55: 83–87

n-3 Fatty acids on autoimmune disease and apoptosis

Gabriel Fernandes

Department of Medicine, Division of Clinical Immunology, The University of Texas Health Science Center at San Antonio, San Antonio, TX 78284-7874, USA

Summary. Source and amount of dietary fat intake modulate cardiovascular disease, malignancy, and autoimmune disorders. Controlled clinical studies reveal *n*-3 fatty acids are able to decrease symptoms and severity of rheumatoid arthritis and systemic lupus erythematosus. Other studies reveal a reduction in the need for anti-inflammatory medications along with significant clinical benefits. When comparing *n*-6 lipid-fed animals with *n*-3 lipid-fed animals, experimental studies indicate *n*-3 lipid exerts its protective effects against autoimmune disorders by enhancing transcriptional activity of various antioxidant enzyme mRNA levels and by decreasing proinflammatory cytokine mRNA expression in the kidney. Results also suggest that a combination of calorie restriction and *n*-3 lipid intake further increase lifespan and also elevate apoptosis by modulating glucocorticoid and Th-1/Th-2 cytokine production. In summary, *n*-3 lipids combined with reduced calorie intake modulate the immune system and gene expression during autoimmunity. Studies exploring the adjustment in *n*-6/*n*-3 fatty acid ratio and its effect on immunity and longevity in both short- and long-lived strains of mice are urgently warranted.

Introduction

Source and level of dietary lipid intake may modulate the onset of autoimmune and cardiovascular diseases (CVD) and certain incidences of cancer. Because saturated fats increase CVD and promote tumor formation, the consumption of polyunsaturated *n*-6 lipids (vegetable fats) has increased in recent years [1] (Fig. 1). Although *n*-6 are found to decrease serum cholesterol levels, they are also found to elevate linoleic (18:2) and arachidonic (20:4) acid levels, which are known to increase synthesis of proinflammatory prostaglandins (E2 series) and leukotrienes. Furthermore, *n*-6 lipids were also found to decrease synthesis of antiinflammatory cytokines, such as interleukin-2 (IL-2) and interferon γ (IFNγ) by T cells. A decrease in IL-2 production accelerates the onset and severity of autoimmune disease by increasing production of autoantibodies by B cells. In contrast, *n*-3 fatty acids from marine oils rich in eicosapentaenoic acid (EPA; 20:5) and docosahexaenoic acid (DHA; 22:6) serve as precursors for prostaglandin E_3 (PGE_3) and leukotrienes-B5 (LTB_5), which prevent platelet aggregation and reduce proinflammatory cytokine levels (IL-1, IL-6, and tumor necrosis factor α (TNFα) [2–5].

Medicinal Fatty Acids in Inflammation, edited by J.M. Kremer

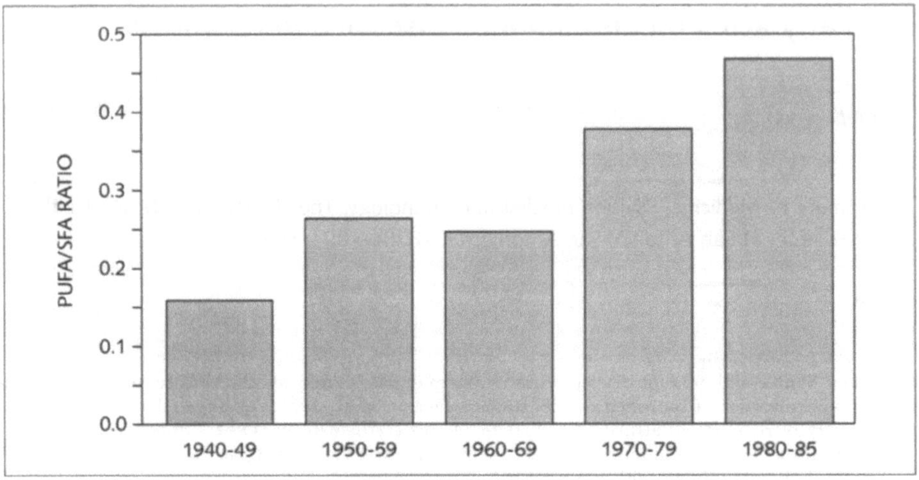

Figure 1
Effect of changes in the consumption of dietary fats on alteration in the ratio of polyunsaturated and saturated fatty acids [1].

Several clinical studies undertaken in patients with active rheumatoid arthritis or systemic lupus erythematosus (SLE) have revealed some level of clinical benefits from the ingestion of fish oil (FO), including a moderate to significant reduction in the usage of antiinflammatory medications [6, 7] (Tab. 1). Earlier studies describing either no benefit or occasionally adverse effects from FO intake are most likely due to the varied sources of marine oils or a failure to supplement FO capsules with adequate antioxidants to prevent rancidity during storage. Also, adequate antioxidant supplements are essential for the prevention of free radical formation during ingestion of FO capsules [8]. Other benefits of FO intake include protection against renal disease induced by formation of immunoglobulin A (IgA) immune complexes. In a multicenter, placebo-controlled, randomized trial, patients taking FO capsules (12 g) with adequate antioxidants showed significant retarded renal disease. At the end of four years, 40% of the patients in the placebo group either died or had end-stage renal disease, whereas 10% of the patients in the FO group had disease ($p = 0.006$). It appears that purified FO with antioxidant supplements may inhibit or delay the progression of renal disease by altering the production of proinflammatory cytokines, growth factors, and prostaglandins including complement, which may decrease antigen deposition and prevent damage to glomeruli and/or renal function [9–16].

During the past three decades, several feeding studies utilizing the *n*-3 fatty acids have shown their ability to block the generation of proinflammatory media-

Table 1 - Beneficial effects of fish oil

In disease state	
Decreases	Increases
Cholesterol, triglycerides	Drug utilization
Severity of autoimmune and cardiovascular diseases	EPA and DHA in phospholipids
Cardiovascular diseases	
Proinflammatory cytokines	
Toxicity of drugs	
Free radical generation	
Oncogene expression	
Transplant rejection	
Blood pressure	
Platelet aggregation	
In normal healthy state	
Useful in infant formula, parenteral feeds, growth, and development	

tors known to be involved in cardiovascular and autoimmune disorders, including asthma, skin disease, and diabetes. Although several animal studies have shown favorable responses from the intake of n-3 fatty acids, in general, human studies have not been as favorable. This is primarily due to the presence of preformed, invisible n-6 fatty acids in various human dietary ingredients. Unless both the visible and invisible sources of dietary n-6 lipids are properly controlled, n-3 fatty acid supplementation may not be as effective in decreasing the precursors of arachidonic acids. Moreover, the use of a proper placebo supplement along with well-controlled dietary fats in a regular diet are essential when comparing the therapeutic value of n-3 fatty acid supplements. Furthermore, a carefully controlled n-6 and n-3 ratio in both human and animal dietary studies is essential when studying the effects on cytokine gene expression and the induction of programmed cell death [17].

In recent years, the role of dietary lipids and gene interaction is receiving greater attention, particularly in the area of cardiovascular disease. At present, several genes are implicated in cholesterol metabolism, which is primarily involved in promoting CVD. It is speculated that n-3 fatty acid downregulates the transcriptional activity of various genes and their products, receptors such as the APOE and low density lipoprotein (LDL) receptors. New insight is now being gained into the mechanism involved in diet and gene interaction by utilizing both transgenic and knockout animal models [18–21].

The effects of *n*-6 and *n*-3 fatty acids on autoimmune disease and gene expression

Studies were undertaken in our laboratory by utilizing a semipurified diet, adding *n*-3 (10%) lipid-rich menhaden FO, fed *ad libitum* to autoimmune lupus-prone NZB/NZW F_1 (B/W) female mice. Results showed a delay in the onset and a slowing of the progression of renal disease as well as a significant lifespan extension compared to mice receiving a *n*-6 lipid-rich corn oil (CO 10%) diet. All diets contained the same level of vitamin E (21.5 mg/100 g). Mice on both FO and CO gained parallel weights (40–45 g); yet, 10% FO in the diet was found to significantly increase the lifespan. Northern blot analysis of kidneys from six month old, FO-fed mice revealed no detectable levels of IL-1β, IL-6, and TNFα mRNA levels, whereas these cytokine mRNAs were easily detected in six month old, CO-fed mice (Fig. 2). In contrast to the cytokine mRNAs, FO-fed mice showed higher renal levels of the antioxidant enzymes catalase (CAT), glutathione peroxidase (GSH-Px), and superoxide dismutase (SOD) mRNAs compared to the CO-fed mice. These results initially suggested that dietary supplementation with a well-defined FO, compared to CO, is likely to inhibit the production of proinflammatory cytokines. This may act to ameliorate immune-complex-mediated kidney injury by enhancing the ability of cells to dispose of harmful reactive oxygen intermediates [22].

We were able to confirm the results of the studies cited above, namely, that the decreased proinflammatory cytokine mRNA levels in kidney tissue of FO-fed mice is due to elevated antioxidant enzyme levels. Therefore, we next set out to compare the effects of *n*-3 lipids on survival and the severity of kidney disease in B/W mice. Furthermore, we compared the hepatic microsomal lipid composition, peroxidation, and the mRNA expression of antioxidant enzymes, such as CAT, GSH-Px, and SOD in 6.5 month old B/W mice. The results revealed [i] significantly higher ($p < 0.001$) CAT, GSH-Px and SOD enzyme activity levels in the liver of B/W mice (Fig. 3); [ii] significantly lower ($p < 0.001$) arachidonic acid (20:4*n*-6) and linoleic acid (12:2*n*-6) levels and higher ($p < 0.001$) EPA (20:5*n*-3) and DHA (22:6*n*-3) levels in hepatic microsomes; and [iii] significantly lower ($p<0.001$) estimated peroxidation indices and thiobarbituric acid reactive substances (TBARS) generation. These findings suggest that one of the mechanisms by which the *n*-3 lipids may delay the onset of autoimmune diseases could be through the maintenance of higher hepatic antioxidant enzyme expression and activity levels [23].

In order to understand the mechanisms involved in promoting renal disease, we decided to also analyze whether transforming growth factor β (TGFβ) plays a pathological role in the induction or progression of glomerulonephritis in B/W mice and whether FO dietary supplementation can modulate the expression of TGFβ. To study this, weanling female B/W mice were divided into three groups. One group was fed an unmanipulated diet (lab chow; LC) and the other two groups were fed a nutritionally adequate, semipurified diet supplemented with 10% CO or FO. Pro-

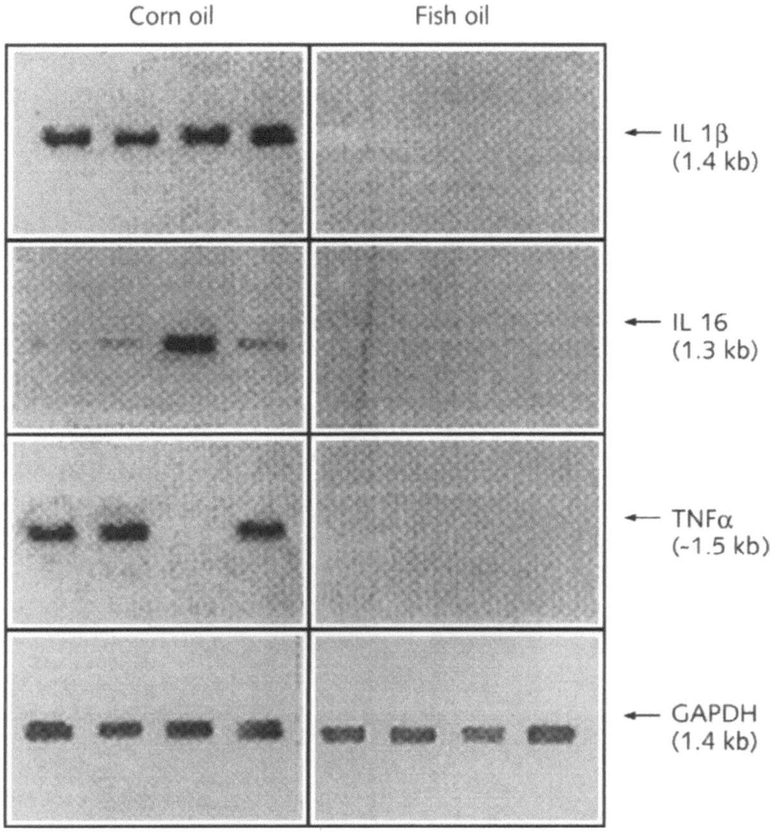

Figure 2
Effects of dietary CO and FO on cytokine mRNA levels in kidneys of B/W mice. Each lane represents mRNA from individual mice [22].

teinuria and serum anti-dsDNA antibody levels were frequently measured to assess disease progression. Mice were killed before the onset of disease at 3.5 months of age, or after the onset of disease at 6.5 months of age. We studied renal mRNA levels for TGFβ isoforms, fibronectin-1 (FN-1), and intercellular adhesion molecule-1 (ICAM-1) using Northern blot analysis. TGFβ1 protein levels were also examined in kidneys by Western blot analysis. The results indicated that at 3.5 months, urinary protein levels were undetectable, very low levels of anti-dsDNA were detected, and no mRNA signal could be detected for the TGFβ isoforms, ICAM-1 and FN-1, in either dietary group. However, at 6.5 months, the FO-fed mice, compared to the

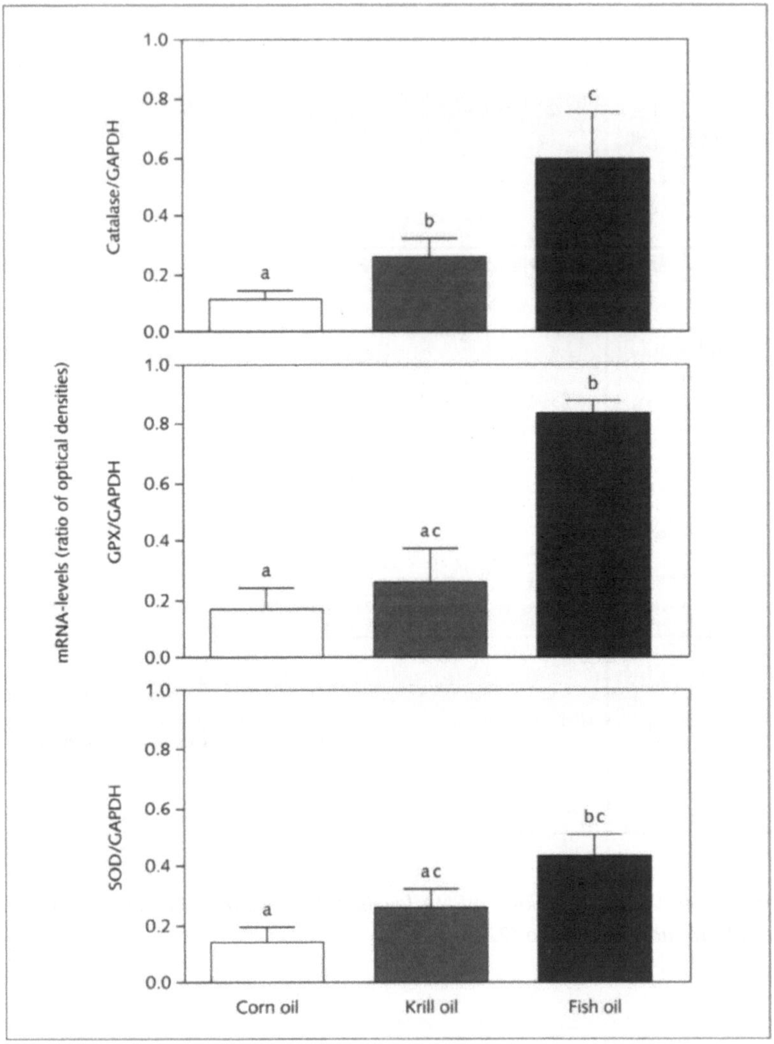

Figure 3
Densitometric analysis of the autoradiographic bands obtained expressed as a ratio of the specific message to the constitutively expressed GAPDH message. The values were tested for significance using the Student's t-test. Values in the figure not denoted by the same superscript are significantly different. The statistical significance of the values tested were as follows: CAT-CO vs. KO: $p<0.05$; $p<0.05$; CO vs. FO; $p<0.01$; KO vs. FO: $p<0.05$; GSH-Px-CO vs. FO: $p<0.01$; KO vs. FO: $p<0.01$; SOD-CO vs. FO: $p<0.01$. CAT, catalase; CO, corn oil; KO, krill oil; FO, fish oil; GSH-Px, glutathione peroxidase; SOD, superoxide dismutase [23].

LC and CO groups, had [i] greatly reduced proteinuria (LC: 2–3+, CO: 2–3+; FO: trace –1+) and serum anti-dsDNA antibodies; [ii] improved survival (50% (8/15) were alive at 12 months (CO: 100% death (15/15) at 8 months)); and [iii] reduced renal TGFβ1 mRNA and protein levels. TGFβ2 and β3 were not significantly affected by the FO diet (Fig. 4). Similarly, lower levels of renal FN-1 and ICAM-1 mRNA were observed in FO-fed mice (Fig. 5). These data indicate that B/W mice fed a FO diet have prolonged survival and amelioration of renal disease, which may be attributed, at least in part, to lower levels of TGFβ1 mRNA and protein in the kidneys [24].

Our next step was to investigate the immune mechanisms by which marine lipids rich in long chain n-3 fatty acids inhibit autoimmune disease in female B/W mice. Again, semipurified diets containing 10% either CO or FO were fed to animals beginning at one month of age and were monitored for proteinuria and survival. In CO-fed mice, proteinuria was detected earlier and became progressively more severe than in the FO-fed mice. The average lifespan was significantly shortened in mice receiving the CO diet (266.7 days ± 12.5). On the other hand, mice receiving the FO diet had significantly increased survival (402.1 days ± 26.1; $p < 0.001$). A cross-sectional study at 6.5 months of age revealed an increased proliferative response to T cell mitogens, including bacterial superantigens and decreased serum anti-dsDNA antibody titers in the FO group compared with the CO group. Furthermore, splenocytes from the FO group, when stimulated with Con A, showed a higher IL-2 and lower IL-4 production, similar to those of young (3.5 month) mice. Flow cytometric analyses of splenocytes revealed lower Ig^+, higher lymphocyte endothelial cell adhesion molecule-1, and lower $Pgp\text{-}1^+$ cells within $CD4^+$ and $CD8^+$ subsets in FO-fed mice. Also, detected in the spleen of FO-fed mice were: elevated IL-2 and IL-4 and significantly higher TGF-β1 levels; lower c-*myc* and c-*ras* mRNA expression; and significantly lower c-Myc and c-Ha-Ras proteins (Fig. 6). Fatty acid analysis of these groups revealed significantly higher linoleic (18:2n-6) and arachidonic (20:4n-6) acid levels in splenocytes of the FO-fed group, but higher EPA (20:5n-3) and DHA (22:6n-3) acid levels in the splenocytes of the CO-fed group, indicating that changes in membrane fatty acid composition of immune cells may contribute to the altered immune function and gene expression during the development of murine SLE [25].

One of the major protective effects of FO is its ability to decrease or prevent the onset of CVD in humans and to ameliorate renal disease in both humans and animals. Indeed, cellular proliferation as an important pathological element in the development of lupus nephritis is well established. We therefore examined the expression of thrombin receptor (TR) and mitogenic agents, such as platelet derived growth factor A (PDGF-A) and -B. Weanling B/W mice were fed either *ad libitum* (AL) or a calorie restricted (CR; 40% less calories than *ad libitum*) diet supplemented with either 5% (w/w) CO or FO. Mice were sacrificed and RNA from renal tissues was extracted from young (3.5–4.0 months of age) before the onset of

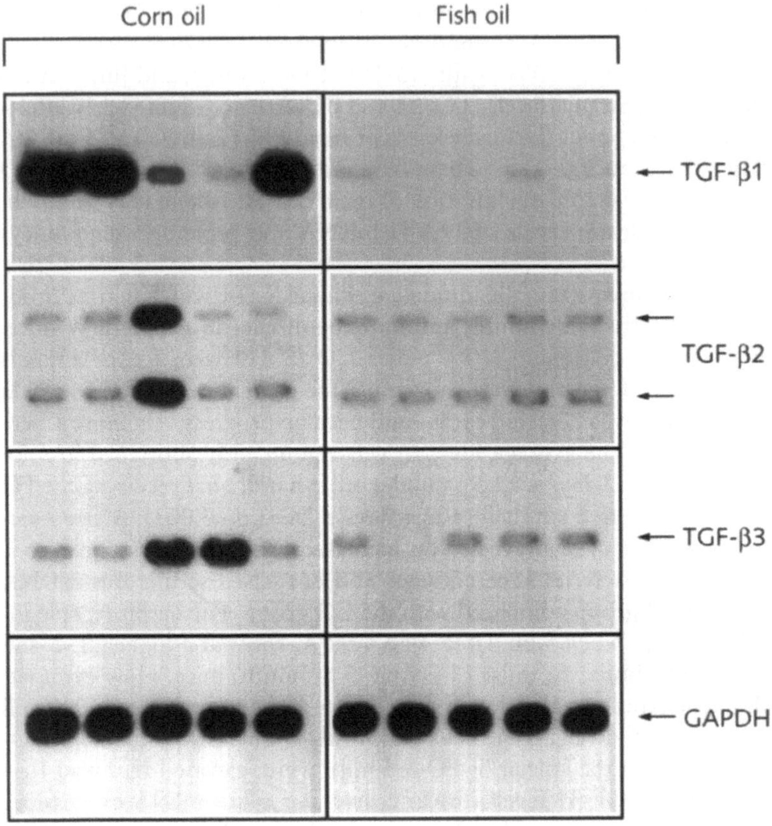

Figure 4
Northern blot analysis of TGFβ isoform mRNA levels: Each lane represents renal RNA from an individual mouse [22].

autoimmune disease and, in old mice (8–10 months of age), after the onset of autoimmune disease. Densitometric analysis (reference gene GAPDH) of blots from Northern analysis (PDGF-A and -B) and ribonuclease protection assay for TR revealed the following results: [i] in young mice, no signal was detected for PDGF-A, -B and TR in all four groups [(1) CO AL, (2) CO CR, (3) FO AL, and (4) FO CR], although the signals were readily detectable in old mice; [ii] in old mice, low and similar levels of PDGF-B were detected – neither CR nor the source of the lipid used altered its expression; [iii] CR significantly inhibited PDGF-A and TR expression in both CO (AL vs CR; PDGF-A, 3.25-fold, $p < 0.025$; TR, 3.7-fold, $p < 0.01$)

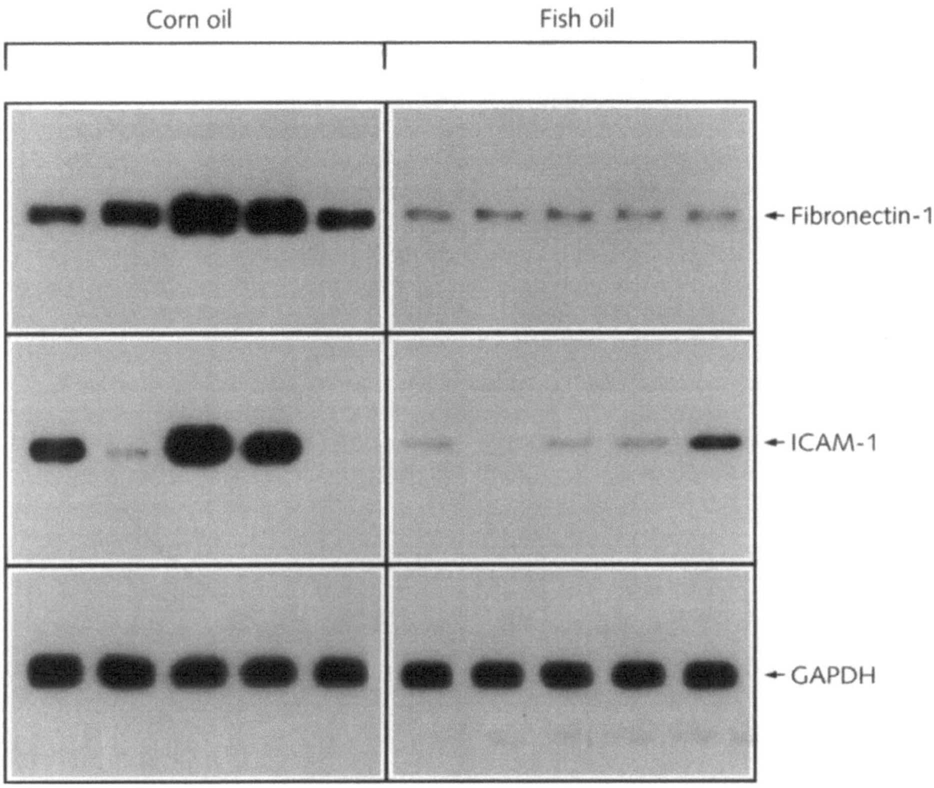

Figure 5
Northern blot analysis of FN-1 and ICAM-1 mRNA levels. Each lane represents renal RNA from an individual mouse [24].

and FO (AL vs CR; PDGF-A, 4.56-fold, $p < 0.01$; TR, 3.6-fold, $p < 0.025$; groups; (iv) although FO (vs CO) produced trends toward decreased expression, results were not statistically significant. We concluded from these studies that the suppression of renal disease in lupus-prone mice by CR is accompanied by decreased expression of PDGF-A and the TR, further confirming the possible beneficial effects of FO on the cardiovascular disease process, as previously noted by several investigators [26].

We also attempted to establish whether restricting dietary calories, in addition to the beneficial effect on kidney disease, could also prevent the salivary gland abnor-

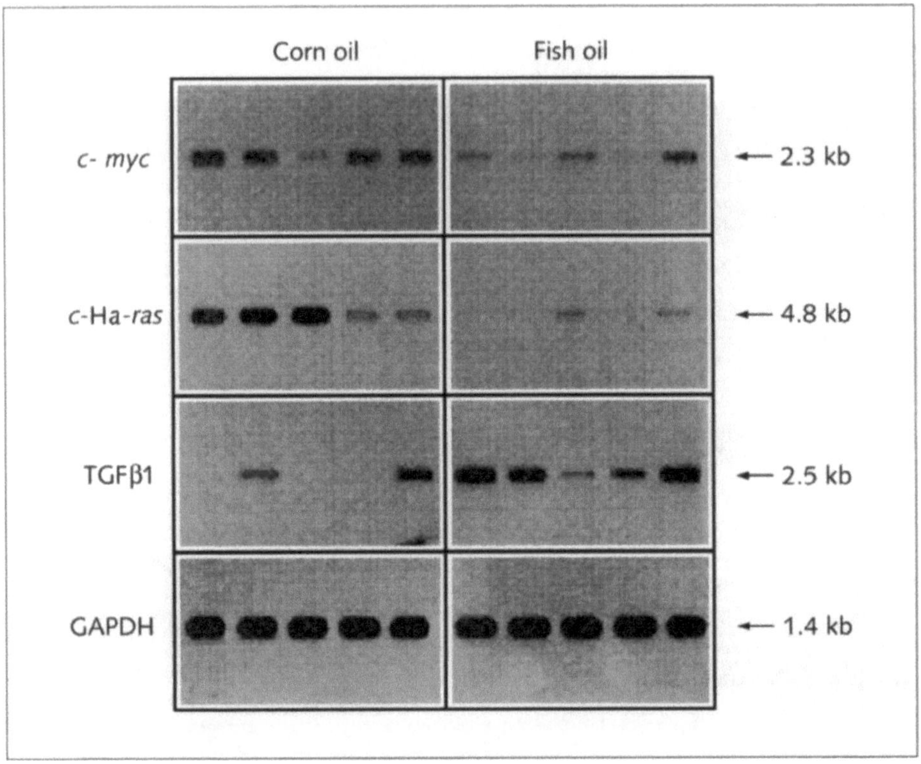

Figure 6
Reduction of oncogene and TGF-β1 mRNA expression by n-3 *lipids. Each lane represents splenic tissue mRNA from an individual mouse [25].*

malities common to B/W mice. We chose to compare the expression of TGFβ and the proinflammatory cytokines, IL-6, and TNFα, in the major salivary glands (SG) of female B/W mice. These mice develop focal lymphocytic interstitial and periductal round cell infiltrates in salivary glands similar to those of humans with Sjögren's syndrome. Both AL and CR fed mice were sacrificed at 3.5 months (young) and 8.5 months (old) of age. Histopathologic and histomorphometric analysis as well as growth factor and cytokine protein and mRNA expression analysis were carried out in the SG. Histomorphometric analysis of SG from young mice showed no differences between AL and CR mice, but old AL (vs old CR) had a 7.3-fold higher focus score and a 34-fold increase in the percentage of area inflammation. Analysis of mRNA revealed significantly higher levels (6.8-fold) of TGFβ1 in the SG of old CR mice. In contrast, CR reduced mRNA expression of proinflammatory cytokines (IL-6, 2.9-fold for young and 4.8-fold for old mice; TNFα, 3.9-fold for old mice). By immunoblotting, significantly higher levels of TGFβ1 protein were detected in old CR mice (vs old AL; 13.2-fold). IL-6 and TNFα proteins were undetectable in both young and old CR groups, whereas an increase in IL-6 (4.7-fold) and TNFα (9.3-fold) was observed in old AL mice. These results indicate that the amelioration of the histological severity of disease in the SG of B/W mice is parallel to and possibly mediated by increased expression of immunosuppressive TGFβ1 and decreased expression of proinflammatory cytokines [27].

Our lipid studies undertaken in short-lived, autoimmune-prone mice indicate that a reduction of proinflammatory cytokines in target tissues, such as the kidney and an elevation of antioxidant enzymes may provide protection against renal disease. However, the role of FO on immune function particularly on T cells as well as the production of various cytokines has not yet been fully analyzed. Our ongoing studies suggest that CR downregulates IL-2 and IFNγ (Th-1 cytokines), whereas in CO and FO AL-fed mice, the Th-1 cytokines are elevated. We do not yet have Th-2 cytokine data for either FO- or CR-fed mice [28].

One of the most paradoxical findings is that FO prolongs the lifespan of short-lived animals, whereas in long-lived strains, it causes immunosuppression (e.g. decreases T cell proliferation and IL-2 production and is suspected to reduce the lifespan due to elevated EPA and DHA fatty acids). This effect may alter co-stimulatory molecules such as CD28 on T cells and B7-1 and B7-2 on antigen-presenting cells differently in short- and long-lived strains of mice. So far, no controlled studies have been carried out to establish the survival rate of non-autoimmune prone, long-lived strains of mice or rats.

Potential mechanism(s): Effect of CR and FO on modulating autoimmunity

CR diet alters glucocorticoid (GC) levels in CR fed mice in a circadian manner, increasing during night time activity and peaking just prior to food intake [29]. Although IL-2 production in AL fed mice is higher than CR fed young mice, CR increases both IL-2 and IL-2R (IL-2Rα, IL-2Rβ and IL-2Rγ) expression in activated lymphocytes of old mice. The increase in IL-2R or TGFβ expression is thought to be driven by glucocorticoids, although conflicting results have been reported [30]. CR also maintains higher weights of both adrenal and thymus glands (relative to body weight) in B/W mice (unpublished data). In addition, there are parallels between the therapeutic effects of glucocorticoids on human lupus nephritis and the amelioration of autoimmune disease by dietary interventions, which are known to elevate glucocorticoids [31].

Glucocorticoid receptor (GCR) responses to stress fall steadily with age, but this decline is attenuated by CR, which is also shown to maintain higher free plasma corticosterone (CORT) levels during aging [32]. Recently, Nelson [33] proposed a hypothesis linking neuroendocrine involvement in the retardation of aging by CR. CR increases CORT levels, particularly during the circadian cycle when both CORT and free CORT levels are elevated. These studies and our results showing elevated Dexamethasone (Dex) stimulated programmed cell death (PCD) in lymphocytes from CR or *n*-3 fed mice led to our new working hypothesis, that *n*-3 and/or CR increases circulating CORT levels and synthesis of CORT in thymic tissue, thereby enhancing negative selection of $CD4^-$,$CD8^-$ (potentially autoreactive) cells [34].

Our pilot data indicated that T cells from CR mice show higher PCD in response to Dex, whereas those from AL mice show higher PCD in response to anti-CD3 antibody. We are attempting to establish that CR maintains higher GC levels and enhances PCD, which facilitates negative selection in the thymus. In contrast, lymphocytes of old AL mice (generally more resistant to differentiation and proliferation *in vivo*) due to anergy of T cells are found more susceptible to PCD induced by anti-CD3. Recent *in vitro* studies with a defined T cell line indicate that T cell receptor (TCR/anti-CD3) -mediated PCD is due to an increased Ca^{2+} influx, followed by activation of endonucleases [35]. In contrast, protein kinase-C (PKC) and/or elevated cytoplasmic cAMP are involved in Dex-induced apoptosis in thymic cells. Thus, the TCR-mediated PCD pathways appear to be separate from the GC or phorbol ester-mediated PCD pathways [36].

We have observed that CR (and other dietary manipulations that increase lifespan) are also associated with increased expression of free radical scavenging enzymes [37]. It is therefore of particular interest to note the connection between free radicals and PCD. Our observations that CR (vs. AL feeding) normalizes PCD to some extent in MRL/*lpr* mice (which have markedly reduced PCD) and increases the expression of *Fas* (a promoter of apoptosis) in B/W mice, supporting the hypothesis that diet can modulate apoptosis in the immune system. Peripheral blood lymphocytes from human patients with SLE showed increased normal PCD activity, which paralleled the severity of clinical symptoms [38]. Although the causes of human SLE may be related to the loss of glucocorticoid levels, these findings, taken together, suggest that dysregulated PCD is an important common denominator in autoimmune disorders. The protective effects of CR appear to be linked to the upregulation of PCD by increasing the activity of GC, whereas increased PCD, independent of GCR, may be the result of the loss of T cell function during autoimmunity.

Modulation of PCD by diet is likely to be particularly relevant to the development of T cells, as 95% of all marrow stem cells transported to the thymus are deleted by PCD and only approximately 5% survive. The unique cellular programs of differentiated T cells, particularly $CD4^+$ and $CD8^+$ T cells, protect the host through release of growth and cytotoxic factors, and their activation, proliferation, and migration to target tissues. Increased loss of immune cells *in vivo* by activated PCD could decrease immunity and lead to increased susceptibility to infection. Alternatively, decreased PCD could cause autoimmune disease and increased rates of malignancy and shortened lifespan. Our current ongoing nutrition and immunity studies are designed to maintain a balanced ratio of Th-1 and Th-2 T cells to produce both anti- and proinflammatory cytokines and to prevent T cell anergy as well as to optimize physiologically maintained glucocorticorticoid-regulated PCD to prevent the early rise of autoimmune disorders with age [28].

Effect of combined FO and CR on autoimmune disease

Although CR alone extends lifespan by decreasing the formation of memory T cells in both short- and long-lived strains of mice or rats [39, 40], our recent observations indicate that FO lipids, containing *n*-3 fatty acids, can further extend life span when combined with CR. In short-lived animals, lifespan was significantly prolonged by replacing CO with FO (10 or 20%) fatty acids even without CR. The combination of *n*-3 and CR significantly increases lifespan in short-lived animals more than CR alone. It is not yet known whether supplementation with *n*-3 fatty acids combined with CR will increase the lifespan of long-lived strains of mice. Furthermore, we observed for the first time, that *n*-3 fatty acids in the presence of antioxidant supplements increase antioxidant enzyme levels. However, we have not yet established whether *n*-3 fatty acid supplement alone, without vitamin E supplementation, increases antioxidant enzyme levels and extends the lifespan. Thus, new studies will be of importance in determining whether *n*-3 supplementation protects against autoimmune disorders by maintaining normal PCD and eliminating the age-related rise of autoreactive cells due to the change in free radical formation.

Products of Bcl-2 and *Fas* genes are important in the regulation of PCD. Bcl-2 was discovered by virtue of its translocation into the Ig locus in B cell lymphomas, which prevented or delayed PCD in response to a number of apoptotic stimuli [41]. Bcl-2 expression is more common in hemopoietic or bone marrow cells, and transgenic mice that constitutively express Bcl-2 more frequently express it in hemopoietic or bone marrow cells. Suppression of PCD is linked to increased Bcl-2 oncogene expression. Constitutive expression of Bcl-2 by B cells in transgenic mice resulted in anti-DNA and anti-Sm autoantibodies and the development of autoimmune renal disease [42].

Fas is the receptor for *Fas* ligand (*Fas*L), a cell death factor. *Fas* (a type I membrane protein) belongs to a receptor supergene family, which includes nerve growth factor, tumor necrosis factor, CD40, and *Fas*L itself [43]. *Fas* is expressed on myeloid and lymphoid cells as well as on fibroblasts, liver cells, heart muscle, and in the ovarian follicle [44]. The cytoplasmic domain of *Fas* probably interacts with signal transduction molecules such as G-proteins, kinases, and/or phospholipases as there is no apparent enzymatic activity associated with *Fas* itself. The recently cloned *Fas*L is a 40 Kd protein expressed on activated splenocytes and cytotoxic T cells [45]. Defective interactions of *Fas* and *Fas*L lead to reduced apoptosis and subsequent induction of autoimmune disease. We recently proposed that either *n*-3 fatty acids and/or calorie restriction may increase negative selection and PCD in the thymus by maintaining higher levels of adrenocorticoids [17]. Maintaining normal physiologically regulated PCD may facilitate the prevention of autoimmune disorders by eliminating the age-associated rise in autoreactive immune cells in the host.

Acknowledgment

This research was partially supported by National Institutes of Health grants AG10531, AG13693, DE10893, AG14541 and by a grant from the Robert J. Kleberg, Jr. and Helen C. Kleberg Foundation at San Antonio.

References

1 Fernandes G, Venkatraman J (1993) Role of ω-3 fatty acids in health and disease. *Nutri Res* 13: S19–S45

2 Calder PC (1995) Fatty acids, dietary lipids and lymphocyte functions. *Biochem Soc Trans* 23: 302–309

3 Calder PC (1996) Immunomodulatory and anti-inflammatory effects of omega-3 polyunsaturated fatty acids. *Proc Nutr Soc* 55: 737–774

4 Calder PC (1997) n-3 polyunsaturated fatty acids and cytokine production in health and disease. *Ann Nutr Metab* 41: 203–234

5 Fritsche KL, Johnston PV (1990) Effect of dietary α-linolenic acid on growth metastasis, fatty acid profile and prostaglandin production of two murine mammary adenocarcinomas. *Nutr Res* 10: 577–588

6 Kremer JM, Bigaquette J, Michalek AV, Timchalk MA, Lininger L, Rynes RI, Huyek C, Zieminski J, Bartholomew LE (1985) Effects of manipulating dietary fatty acids on clinical manifestations of rheumatoid arthritis. *Lancet* i: 184–187

7 Kremer JM, Jubiz W, Michalek A, Rynes RI, Bartholomew LE, Bigaquette J, Timchalk M, Beeler D, Lininger L (1987) Fish oil fatty acid supplementation in active rheumatoid arthritis. A double-blinded, controlled, crossover study. *Ann Int Med* 106: 497–502

8 Fernandes G, Venkatraman J, Troyer DA (1996) Interaction of Vitamin E with n-6 and n-3 polyunsaturated fatty acids. *Int Soc Study Fatty Acids & Lipids* 3: 10–13

9 DeCaterina R, Caprioli R, Giannessi D, Sicari R, Galli C, Lazzarini G, Bernini W, Carr L, Rindi P (1993) n-3 fatty acids reduced proteinuria in patients with chronic glomerulonephritis. *Kid Int* 49: 603–607

10 DeCaterina R, Endres S, Kristensen SD, Schmidt EB (1994) n-3 fatty acids and renal diseases. *Am J Kid Dis* 24: 397–415

11 Donadio JVJ, Bergstralh EJ, Offord KP, Spencer DC, Holley KE (1994) A controlled

trial of fish oil in IgA nephropathy. Mayo Nephrology Collaborative Group. *NEJM* 331: 1194–1199

12 Gentile MG, Fellin G, Cofano F, Delle Fave A, Mannan G, Iciceri R, Petrini C, Lavarda F, Pozzi F, D'Amico G (1993) Treatment of proteinuric patients with a vegetarian soy diet and fish oil. *Clin Nephrol* 40: 315–320

13 Lin C (1994) Treatment of IgA nephropathy. *Springer Semin Immunopathol* 16: 121–127

14 Morphake P, Briety J, Darlametsos I, Tsipas G, Gkikas G (1994) Alteration of cyclosporine (CsA-induced nephrotoxicity by gamma linolenic acid (GLA) and eicosapentaenoic acid (EPA) in Winstar rats. *Prostaglandins Leukot Essent Fatty Acids* 50: 29–35

15 Nordkild PK, Graff J, Jorgensen HE, Fugleberg S (1993) Fish oil and antioxidant supplements reduce erythropoietin requirement in haemodialysis patients. *Nephrol Dialysis Transplant* 8: 569

16 Pettersson EE, Rekola S, Berglund L, Sundqvist KG, Angelin B, Diczfalusy U, Bjorkhem I, Bergstrom J (1994) Treatment of IgA nephropathy with omega-3-polyunsaturated fatty acids: a prospective, double-blind, randomized study. *Clin Nephrol* 41: 183–190

17 Troyer D, Fernandes G (1996) Nutrition and apoptosis. *Nutr Res* 16: 1959–1988

18 Clarke SD, Jump DB (1994) Dietary polyunsaturated fatty acid regulation of gene transcription. *Ann Rev Nutri* 14: 83–98

19 Fernandes G, Chandrasekar B, Troyer DA, Venkatraman JT, Good RA (1995) Dietary lipids and calorie restriction affect mammary tumor incidence and gene expression in mouse mammary tumor virus/v-Ha-*ras* transgenic mice. *Proc Natl Acad Sci USA* 92: 6494–6498

20 Niot I, Poirier H, Bezard PH (1997) Regulation of gene expression by fatty acids: special reference to fatty acid-binding protein (FABP). *Biochimie* 79: 129–133

21 Willumsen N, Vaagenes H, Lie O, Rustan AC, Berge RK (1996) Eicosapentaenoic acid, but not docosahexaenoic acid, increases mitochrondial fatty acid oxidation and upregulated 2,4-dienoyl-CoA reductase gene expression in rats. *Lipids* 31: 579–592

22 Chandrasekar B, Fernandes G (1994) Decreased pro-inflammatory cytokines and increased antioxidant enzyme gene expression by ω-3 lipids in murine lupus nephritis. *Biochem Biophy Res Com* 200: 893–898

23 Venkatraman JT, Chandrasekar B, Kim JD, Fernandes G (1994) Effects of n-3 and n-6 fatty acids on the activities and expression of hepatic antioxidant enzymes in autoimmune-prone NZBxNZW F1 mice. *Lipids* 29: 561–567

24 Chandrasekar B, Troyer DA, Venkatraman JT, Fernandes G (1995) Dietary omega-3 lipids delay the onset and progression of autoimmune lupus nephritis by inhibiting transforming growth factor-beta mRNA and protein expression. *J Autoimmunity* 8: 381–393

25 Fernandes G, Chandrasekar B, Venkatraman J, Tomar V, Zhao W (1994) Increased TGFβ and decreased oncogene expression by ω-3 lipids in the spleen delays autoimmune disease in B/W mice. *J Immunol* 152: 5979–5987

26 Troyer DA, Chandrasekar B, Barnes JL, Fernandes G (1997) Calorie restriction decreases platelet-derived growth factor (PDGF)-A and thrombin receptor mRNA expression in autoimmune murine lupus nephritis. *Clin Exp Immunol* 108: 58–62
27 Chandrasekar B, McGuff HS, Aufdemorte TB, Troyer DA, Talal N, Fernandes G (1995) Effects of calorie restriction on transforming growth factor-beta-1 and proinflammatory cytokines in murine Sjögren's syndrome. *Clin Immun & Immunopath* 76: 291–296
28 Fernandes G, Jolly CA (1998) Nutrition and autoimmune disease. *Nutrition Reviews* 56: S161–S169
29 Sabatini F, Masoro EJ, McMahan CA, Kuhn RW (1991) Assessment of the role of the glucorticoid system in aging processes and in the action of food restriction. *J Gerontol Biol Sci* 46: B171–B179
30 Gillis S, Crabtree GR, Smith KA (1979) Glucocorticoid induced inhibition of T cell growth factor production. I. The effect of mitogen-induced lymphocyte proliferation. *J Immunol* 123: 1624–1631
31 Chikanza IC, Petrou P, Kingsley G, Chrousos G, Panayi GS (1992) Defective hypothalamicresponse to immune and inflammatory stimuli in patients with rheumatoid arthritis. *Arthritis & Rheumatism* 35: 1281–1288
32 Sapolsky RM, Krey LC, McEwen BS (1986) The neuroendocrinology of stress and aging: The glucocorticoid cascade hypothesis. *Endocrin Rev* 7: 284–301
33 Nelson JF (1992) The potential role of endocrine systems in the retardation of aging by caloric restriction. *Age Nutr* 3: 171–178.
34 Wilder RL (1995) Neuroendocrine-immune system interactions and autoimmunity. *Annu Rev Immunol* 13: 307–338
35 Hoshi S, Furntani-Seiki M, Seto M, Tada T, Asaro Y (1989) Prevention of TCR-mediated apoptosis by the elevation of cAMP. *Int Immunol* 6: 1081–1089
36 Oshimi Y, Mayazaki S (1995) Fas antigen-mediated DNA fragmentation and apoptotic morphologic changes are regulated by elevated cytosolic Ca^{2+} level. *J Immunol* 154: 599–609
37 Byun DS, Venkatraman J, Yu B, Fernandes G (1995) Modulation of antioxidant activities and immune response by food restriction in aging Fischer-344 rats. *Aging Clin Expt* Res 7: 40–48
38 Emlen W, Niebur J, Kadera R (1994) Accelerated *in vitro* apoptosis of lymphocytes from patients with systemic lupus erythematosus. *J Immunol* 152: 3685–3692
39 Venkatraman JT, Attwood VG, Turturro A, Hart RW, Fernandes G (1994) Maintenance of virgin T cells and immune functions by food restriction during aging in long-lived B6D2F1 female mice. *Aging, Immunol & Infect Dis* 5: 13–25
40 Fernandes G, Venkatraman J, Turturro A, Attwood VG, Hart RW (1997) Effect of food restriction on life span and immune functions in long-lived Fischer-344 X Brown Norway F1 rats. *J Clin Immunol* 17: 85–95
41 Hawkins CJ, Vaux DL (1994) Analysis of the role of bcl-2 in apoptosis. *Immunol Rev* 142: 127–139
42. Strasser A, Senga W, Vaux DL, Bath ML, Adams CS, Harris AW (1991) Enforced Bcl-2

expression in B-lymphoid cells prolongs antibody responses and elicits autoimmune disease. *Proc Natl Acad Sci USA* 88: 8661–8665

43 Itoh N, Tsujimoto Y, Nagata S (1993) Effect of bcl-2 *Fas* antigen-mediated cell death. *J Immunol* 151: 621–627

44 Watanabe-Fukunaga R, Brannan CI, Copeland NG, Jenkins NA, Nagata S (1992) Lymphoproliferative disorder in mice explained by defects in *fas* antigen that mediates apoptosis. *Nature* 356: 314–317

45 Takahashi T, Tanaka M, Inazawa J, Abe T, Suda T, Nagata S (1994) Human Fas ligand: Gene structure, chromosomal location and species specificity. *Int Immunol* 6: 1567–1574

n-3 Fatty acids in the treatment of Crohn's disease

Andrea Belluzzi and Federico Miglio

Department of Emergency Medicine, S. Orsola Hospital, Via Massarenti, 9, I-40138 Bologna, Italy

Overview

Crohn's disease (CD) is an idiopathic inflammatory bowel disease that may have pathological and clinical manifestations in any part of the alimentary tract from the mouth to the anus, but mainly in the ileum and in the colon. The etiology and the pathogenesis are as yet unknown, but several observations suggest that, as in other chronic inflammatory processes, the pathogenesis of the inflammation can be divided in two stages.

The first stage is the initiating event which triggers the inflammatory response, as yet unknown in CD, and the second stage is the amplification of the inflammatory response which involves a number of inflammatory cells including lymphocytes, mastcells, macrophages, neutrophils and soluble mediators such as eicosanoids, several cytokines as well as bacterial product formyl methionine leucine phenylalanine (FMLP), neuropeptides and free radicals.

The rationale for n-3 fatty acids (n-3 FAs) supplementation in the gastrointestinal tract resides in broad anti-inflammatory effects of these lipid compounds shown in the last 15 years, and one of the first lines of evidence of the importance of dietary intake of n-3 polyunsaturated fatty acids was derived from epidemiological observations regarding the very low incidence of inflammatory bowel disease in people eating large amount of fish, a great source of n-3 FAs, such as Greenland Eskimos [1].

The n-3 FAs act by lowering the production of the most active arachidonic acid (AA) metabolite, leukotriene B_4 [2], which is elevated in inflamed intestinal mucosa [3], along with a reduction in another AA metabolite, thromboxane A_2, which is released in uninflamed mucosa in CD, as an early abnormality of special pathogenic significance [4].

It has also been demonstrated [5] that dietary supplementation of n-3 FAs can inhibit interleukin-1 beta and tumor necrosis factor production, and that inhibition lasted several days after the end of supplementation; the decreased production of interleukin-1 and tumor necrosis factor was also accompanied by a decreased ratio

Medicinal Fatty Acids in Inflammation, edited by J.M. Kremer

of AA to eicosapentaenoic acid (EPA) in the membrane phospholipids. It has been also shown that *n*-3 FAs can act as free-radical scavengers [6].

Moreover, multifocal gastrointestinal infarctions have been suggested as one of the first pathogenic steps in CD [7], thus suggesting a pivotal role for platelets and for the powerful platelet aggregator thromboxane A_2, and giving an explanation to the increased frequency of thromboembolic complications observed in patients with CD [8]. Treatment with *n*-3 FAs was able to reverse increased platelet responsiveness, and to restore the platelets sensitivity to a stable prostacyclin analogue, that is impaired in patients with CD [9].

Finally, it has been demonstrated that fish oil supplementation improves the nutritional state of rats in which a short bowel syndrome was induced. These results were obtained by inducing enterocyte hyperplasia, which markedly increases the mucosal surface area with a corresponding increase in enteral absorption [10].

The first prospective, controlled and double-blind study was published by Lorenz [11] who treated 39 patients with inflammatory bowel disease, of which 29 had CD in different stages of clinical activity, in a 7 months controlled crossover trial. Patients were randomised to receive either 3.2 g daily of *n*-3-FAs or olive oil as placebo. Conventional treatment was discontinued whenever possible. Otherwise it was minimised and kept constant for at least 3 weeks before the study and until completion. There was 1 month washout period between the two treatments.

At the end of the study, the clinical activity, expressed by Crohn's Disease Activity Index (CDAI), of CD patients was unchanged by *n*-3 FAs supplementation. This index [12] incorporates eight items – the daily number of liquid or very soft stools, abdominal pain, general well-being, extraintestinal manifestations of CD, use of opiates to treat diarrhoea, abdominal mass, hematocrit and body weight – to yield a composite score ranging from 0 to 600. Higher scores indicate more disease activity. Patients with CDAI scores of 150 or less are considered to have inactive disease.

It is also very important to consider that in this study, the crossover design, characterised by a very short washout period between the two treatments, did not allow a complete displacement of the extra 3-FAs from the membrane and therefore could have interfered with the final results of the studies, since it has been demonstrated that a biological effect of *n*-3 FAs, i.e. inhibition of cytokine production, lasts for more than 10 weeks after the suspension of *n*-3 FAs [5].

Mate et al. [13] reported preliminary data on a group of 38 CD patients in clinical and laboratory remission, characterised by a CDAI < 150. The patients were randomly separated into two groups: group a, 19 patients who were put on placebo; and group b, 19 patients who received a diet with high content of fish oil (from 100 to 250 g of fish daily) for 2 years. At the end of the study, 6 patients in group a and 4 in group b left the trial; amongst patients who ended the study, 7 of 13 relapsed (54%) in the placebo group and 3 of 15 relapsed (20%) in the fish oil group. Thus, those receiving the enriched *n*-3 FAs diet seem to have prolonged remission.

More recently Lorenz-Meyer et al. [14] published data from a large placebo controlled trial in 204 CD patients. Patients were included after an acute relapse of their disease in which remission (CDAI < 150) was obtained under steroid therapy. Patients were randomised to receive either *n*-3 FAs with 5.1 g/day fish oil in the chemical form of ethylesters (n = 70), or a carbohydrate-reduced diet, 72 g/day (n = 69) or placebo (n = 65), for 1 year. A low dosage of prednisolone was given to all patients for the first 8 weeks of the trial and then discontinued.

On an intent-to-treat analysis none of the treatments were able to prevent a clinical flare-up, but the diet poor in carbohydrates, although containing the highest numbers of dropouts [20 on 69 (35%)], seemed to be effective ($p < 0.05$).

It is very important to mention that the CD population of this interesting study represents a big challenge for gastroenterologists: it is well known that CD patients treated with steroids for an acute flare-up of the disease have more than a 60% likelihood of relapsing in a 6 months period, after the steroid suspension [15] and they often become steroid-dependent. Due to the strong side effects of steroids in long term treatment, most of these patients are shifted to an immunosuppressant treatment, the most potent class of drugs available for treating CD.

Some criticisms can be raised on the choice of placebo. In both studies [11, 14] the placebo was olive oil and due to its content of phenols, may exert some important beneficial effects, such as free radical scavenger properties [16] and inhibition of eicosanoid formation [17,18], and may have interfered with the final end-point of these two trials.

In many of the studies in which high doses of fish oil have been used, poor patient compliance was registered [19–21]. This was induced by poor palatability and by minor, but very annoying side effects such as halitosis, belching and diarrhoea, related to the high daily intake of fish oil preparations necessary for obtaining a satisfactory intestinal absorption and incorporation of 3-FAs into membranes.

Moreover two recent studies have compared the intestinal absorption of 3 different chemical formulations of fish oil, triacylglicerol, ester, and free fatty acids, showing that absorption of the dose administered was, respectively, 60%, 20% and 95%. The better absorption of the free fatty acid formulation may be due to its ability to cross the intestinal wall without necessitating the enzymatic cleavage operated by lipases, the availability of which could be a limiting factor in the absorption of the other chemical formulations, namely ethyl esters or triacylglicerol derivatives [22, 23].

For these reasons we decided to carry out a study of patient tolerance in a group of CD patients with a new *n*-3 mixture FAs, consisting of 500 mg (40%) eicosapentaenoic acid (EPA) and 20% docosahexaenoic acid (DHA) (20%) as free fatty acids in enteric coated (gastric-resistant) capsules, in comparison with traditional *n*-3 FAs which are in the form of triacylglicerols.

The patients were randomized into five groups of 10 patients each and supplemented with four different Purepa preparations (EPA 40%, DHA 20%, Tillotts-Pharma, Ziefen, Switzerland): (A) uncoated Purepa; (B) Purepa, pH 5.5, with cellulose acetate trimellitate coating (CAT); (C) Purepa, pH 5.5, 60 min time release with CAT coating; (D) Purepa, pH 6.9, with cellulose acetate phthalate coating (CAP); (E) triglyceride fish oil preparation (EPA 18%, DHA 10%) (Tab. 1).

The incorporation of *n*-3 FAs into phospholipids in plasma, as well as in red cell membranes, has been evaluated. We have found that the absorption rate of *n*-3 fatty acids is high when they are administered as free fatty acids in enteric coated preparation (group C), the dose needed to achieve the incorporation into phospholipid membranes is one-third of the dose used previously. As a result, the frequency of side effects is reduced, compliance is increased, and long-term treatment becomes feasible in many patients (Tab. 2) [24].

Table 1 - Percentage of arachidonic, eicosapentaenoic and docosahexaenoic acids incorporated into red blood cells (A), and plasma phospholipid membranes (B), before and after six weeks of treatment in five different groups of Crohn's disease patients.

A

Fatty acids (%)	**Group A**		**Group B**		**Group C**		**Group D**		**Group E**	
Δ (after-before)	**before**	**after**	**before**	**after**	**before**	**after**	**before**	**after**	**before**	**after**
Arachidonic	17.5	15.5	18.0	16.0	17.8	13.2	18.1	17.7	18.1	17.0
Δ	−2		−2		−4.6		−0.4		−1.1	
Eicosapentaenoic	0.2	2.4	0.3	2.8	0.2	4.4	0.4	1.1	0.4	1.4
Δ	+2.2		+2.5		+4.2		+0.7		+1	
Docosaehexaenoic	3.5	5.0	3.4	4.9	3.7	6.3	3.2	4.0	3.2	4.2
Δ	+1.5		+1.5		+2.6		+0.8		+1	

B

Fatty acids (%)	**Group A**		**Group B**		**Group C**		**Group D**		**Group E**	
Δ (after-before)	**before**	**after**	**before**	**after**	**before**	**after**	**before**	**after**	**before**	**after**
Arachidonic	7.9	6.1	9.1	7.8	8.5	6.1	8.8	6.5	8.4	6.8
Δ	−0.2		−1.2		−2.4		−2.3		−1.6	
Eicosapentaenoic	0.4	4.8	0.5	4.2	0.5	8.5	0.6	2.8	0.55	3.2
Δ	+4.4		+3.7		+8		+2.2		+2.65	
Docosaehexaenoic	2.3	4.1	1.9	4.0	2.4	5.3	2.8	3.6	2.0	3.7
Δ	+1.8		+2.1		+2.9		+1.8		+1.7	

From Belluzzi et al. [24]

We performed a one year double-blind placebo controlled study to investigate the effect of this new free fatty acid formulation in the maintenance of remission in 78 CD patients who had high risk of relapsing. It is well known that, since CD is characterised by remission and clinical relapse, a short previous remission and/or alteration of acute phase proteins appear to indicate a high risk of flare-up [25-27].

Outpatients were assessed to determine whether they satisfied all of the following criteria:

- Crohn's Disease Activity Index < 150 for at least 3 months but less then 2 years;
- at least one abnormal value of alpha-1 acid glycoprotein > 130 mg per decilitre (reference range < 120 mg per decilitre); erythrocyte sedimentation rate > 40 mm per hour (reference range < 20 mm per hour); alpha-2 globulin > 0.9 g per decilitre (reference range < 0.8 g per decilitre);
- no treatment with 5-aminosalicylate, sulphasalazine or corticosteroids in previous 3 months, or with immunosuppressive therapy in previous 6 months;
- if patients already operated upon, documentation of clinical and endoscopical or radiological recurrence with subsequent remission, after surgery;
- no previous bowel resection > 1 metre;
- age 18–75 years.

Of 89 potentially eligible patients, 78 were enrolled in the study. The reasons for exclusion were unwillingness to participate in the study (5 patients), pregnancy or a desire to become pregnant (3 patients) and the impossibility to attend follow-up visits (3 patients).

The fish oil capsules used were 500 mg of a new marine lipid concentrate in free fatty acid form containing 40% EPA and 20% DHA. The capsules were coated to resist gastric acid for at least 30 minutes and to disintegrate within 60 minutes, possibly allowing release of fish oil into the small intestine.

Table 2 - Side effects registered in 50 patients with Crohn's disease treated with 5 different types of fish oil preparations

	Patients compliance				
	Group A	**Group B**	**Group C**	**Group D**	**Group E**
Total patient number	10	10	10	10	10
Upper GI (belching, flatulance, halitosis, etc)	5	0	0	0	6
Lower GI (increased bowel motions)	0	5	0	7	2
No side effects	5	5	10	3	2

From Belluzzi et al. [24]

Each patient was randomly given 3 enteric-coated capsules of fish oil three times daily or 3 enteric-coated capsules of identical appearance containing 500 mg of placebo three times daily (Miglyol 812, a mixed acid triglyceride of fractionated fatty acids: 60% capryl acid and 40% capric acid.

Patients on active treatment received 1.8 g of EPA and 0.9 g of DHA daily, for 12 months. All participants were examined on entry to the study and at 3, 6, 9 and 12 months, or before if symptoms worsened. Relapse was defined as an increase of Crohn's Disease Activity Index of at least 100 points over baseline value, and above 150 for more than 2 weeks. At each visit, routine laboratory tests including blood cell count, creatinine, liver function, erythrocyte sedimentation rate, alpha-1 acid glycoprotein, and alpha-2 globulins were performed. At the beginning, 6 months and at the end of the study, 2 ml of packed red cells were obtained and fatty acid phospholipid profile was identified by gas-chromatography.

In the fish oil group, 1 patient withdrew (moved away) and 4 dropped out because of diarrhoea. In the placebo group, 1 patient withdrew (did not attend the outpatient clinic) and 1 dropped out because of diarrhoea. Diarrhoea began in all 5 cases within the first month of treatment and symptoms did not improve when the daily capsule intake was reduced. No other side effects were registered.

Among the 39 patients in the *n*-3 fatty acid group, 11 (28%) had relapses, in contrast, 27 of 39 patients (69%) in the placebo group had relapses ($p < 0.001$). After one year, 23 patients (59%) in the *n*-3 FA group remained in remission, as compared with 10 (26%) in the placebo group ($p = 0.003$). Logistic-regression analysis indicated that only *n*-3 FAs and not sex, age, previous surgery, duration of disease, or smoking status affected the likelihood of relapse (Fig. 1) [28].

The changes in the levels of the main fatty acids in the patients still in remission at the end of the study, indicated a remarkable incorporation of *n*-3 fatty acids in the phospholipid membranes of patients given fish oil, by displacing almost completely the AA (Tab. 3).

No significant differences were found in disease distribution of patients given fish oil who relapsed (ileum = 8, ileum + colon = 6; colon = 1).

Since CD patients frequently require surgery for complications such as strictures, fistulas and abscesses, we recently carried out a new placebo controlled trial in CD patients who underwent surgical gut resection [29]. The percentage of patients whose ileal region is involved and who have undergone surgery 10 years after the first symptoms appeared, is 86% [30, 31].

Unfortunately resection does not offer cure, and 73–93% of cases show reappearance of new lesions well documented by endoscopy within 1 year after surgery, and in 34–86%, subsequent clinical relapse is described to occur within 3 years [32–33].

In a one year double-blind placebo controlled study, 50 patients were treated with 9 capsules of this new *n*-3 fatty acid preparation containing a total of 2.7 g of free fatty acids ($n = 26$), or 9 placebo capsules ($n = 24$), within 1 month after ileal

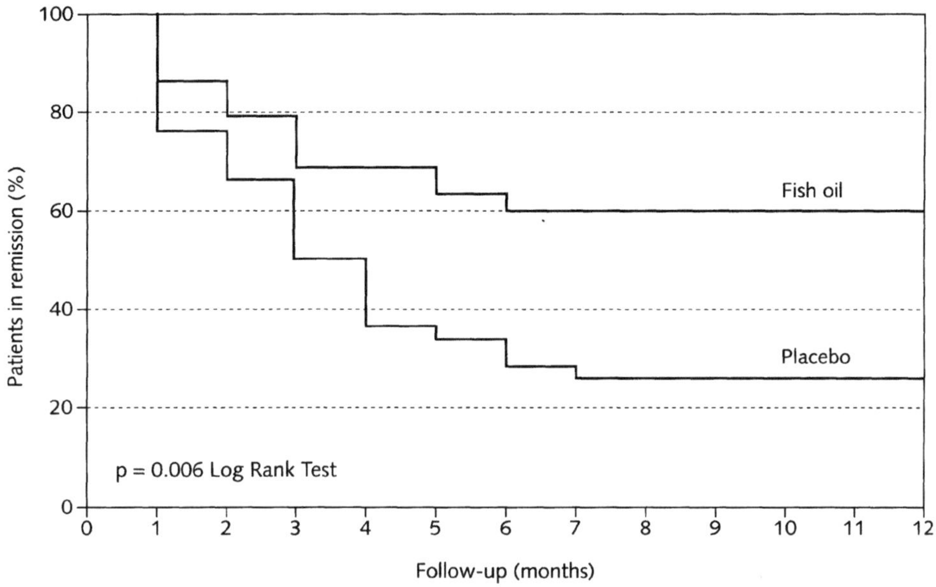

Figure 1
Life-table curves for patients remaining in clinical remission (from Belluzzi et al., with permission).

resection. After 12 months of treatment, severity of endoscopic lesions was recorded with a five-point score as suggested by Rutgeerts [33]; if it was not possible to reach the anastomosis by endoscopy, a barium enema was performed. The results showed seven clinical relapses (2 in the *n*-3 fatty acid group) and 8 drop-outs (4 in the *n*-3 fatty acid group). After 12 months, the rate of severe endoscopic recurrences (score 3–4) was 25% (4/16) in the *n*-3 fatty acid group vs 53% (8/15 in the placebo group) (chi-square 2.6; p value not significant); the overall rate of severe recurrence (score 3–4 on endoscopy or radiological documentation) on "per-protocol" analysis was 23% (5/22) in the *n*-3 fatty acid group vs 55% (11/20) in the placebo group (chi-square 4.6; $p = 0.03$ difference 32%: 95% confidence interval, 7-57) and on "intent-to-treat" analysis was 34% (9/26) in *n*-3 fatty acid group versus 62% (15/24) in the placebo group (chi-square 3.8; $p = 0.04$ difference 28%, 95% confidence interval, 2–54). Logistic-regression analysis indicated that among sex, age, previous surgery, duration of disease and smoking status, only the *n*-3 fatty acid preparation affected the likelihood of relapse (chi-square 3.75; $p = 0.05$) [29].

This review of the literature concerning the use of *n*-3 fatty acids in CD underlines results that seem to be rather controversial. The reasons for the discrepancies

Table 3 - Changes in the levels of the main fatty acids in red blood cells of patients in remission at the end of the study

	Placebo ($n = 39$)	**Fish oil ($n = 39$)**
Linoleic acid (C18:2, *n*-6)		
Base line	10.6 ± 0.5	10.2 ± 0.5
End of study	11.1 ± 0.5	6.4 ± 0.1
% Change (95% CI)	+1 (2.1 to 3.9)	–40 (–14 to –65)*
Arachidonic acid (C20:4, *n*-6)		
Base line	13.5 ± 0.4	13.9 ± 0.3
End of study	14.1 ± 0.3	7.1 ± 0.2
% Change (95% CI)	+0.5 (–3.4 to 4)	-48 (–20 to –76)*
Eicosapentaenoic acid (C20:5, *n*-3)		
Base line	0.3 ± 0.03	0.2 ± 0.02
End of study	0.2 ± 0.03	5.8 ± 0.1
% Change (95% CI)	–3 (–13 to 7)	+2800 (2632 to 3068)*
Docosahexaenoic acid (C22:6, *n*-3)		
Base line	3.2 ± 0.1	2.9 ± 0.1
End of study	3 ± 0.2	11.4 ± 0.2
% Change (95% CI)	–7 (–23 to 9)	+360 (287 to 443)*

Values are means (%) ± SE. CI denotes confidence interval. Changes are percent (95% CI)
*Mann-Whitney U-test for changes in placebo vs fish oil; * = $p < 0.001$*
From Belluzzi et al. [28]

could reside in different study design as well as in various formulations and dosages which could lead to a very high incidence of side effects. It is possible that the *n*-3 FAs act by treating low-grade active inflammation, rather than by preventing reinitiation of the disease process from a truly quiescent state. Whether this treatment is applicable to all CD patients has not been fully elucidated. Epidemiological evidence concerning the incidence of CD in Japan have recently shown that increasing incidence of CD was strongly correlated to the ratio of *n*-6 to *n*-3 fatty acids intake ($r = 0.792$), as demonstrated by Shoda et al. [34], who suggested that increased dietary intake of *n*-6 polyunsaturated fatty acids and less *n*-3 polyunsaturated fatty acids, may contribute to the development of CD.

In conclusion, the importance of the formulation in lowering the incidence of side effects along with a careful selection of patients and experimental design seems to emphasise the therapeutic potential of these lipids in the therapy of CD.

References

1 Bang HO, Dyberg J and Hjorne N (1976) The composition of food consumed by Greenland Eskimos. *Acta Med Scan* 200: 69–73

2 Lee TH, Hoover RL, Williams D, Sperling RI, Ravalese III J, Spur BW, Robinson DR, Corey EJ, Lewis RA and Austen KF (1985) Effect of dietary enrichment with eicosapentaenoic acid and docosahexaenoic acids on *in vitro* polymorphonuclear and monocyte leukotriene generation and polymorphonuclear leukocyte function. *N Engl J Med* 312: 1217–1224

3 Sharon P, Stenson WF (1984) Enhanced synthesis of leukotriene B4 by colonic mucosa in inflammatory bowel disease. *Gastroenterology* 86: 453–460.

4 Rampton DS, Collins CE (1993) Review article: thromboxanes in inflammatory bowel disease-pathogenic and therapeutic implications. *Aliment Pharm and Therap* 7: 357–367

5 Endres S, Ghorbani R, Kelly VE, Georgilis K, Lonnemann G, Van der Meer JWM, Cannon JG, Rogers TS, Klempner MS, Weber PC et al (1989) The effect of dietary supplementation with *n*-3 fatty acids on the synthesis of interleukin-1 and tumor necrosis factor by mononuclear cells. *N Engl J Med* 320: 265–270

6 Fisher M, Upchurch KS, Levine PH, Johnson MH, Vaudreuil CH, Natale A, Hoogasian JJ (1986) Effect of dietary fish oil supplementation on polymorphonuclear leucocyte inflammatory potential. *Inflammation* 10: 387–391.

7 Wakefield AJ, Sankey EA, Dhillon AP, Sawyerr AM, More L, Sim R, Pitillo RM, Rowles PM, Hudson M, Lewis AA et al (1991) Granulomatous vasculitis in Crohn's disease. *Gastroenterology* 100: 1272–1287

8 Webberley MJ, Hart MT, Melikian V (1993) Thromboembolism in inflammatory bowel disease: role of platelets. *Gut* 34: 247–251

9 Jaschoenek K, Clemens MR, Scheurlen M (1991) Decreased responsiveness of platelets to a stable prostacyclin analogue in patients with Crohn's disease. Reversal by *n*-3 polyunsaturated fatty acids. *Thromb Res* 63: 667–672

10 Vanderhoof JA, Park JHY, Herrington MK, Adrian TE (1994) Effects of dietary menhaden oil mucosal adaptation after small bowel resection in rats. *Gastroenterology* 106: 94–99

11 Lorenz R, Weber PC, Szimnau P, Heldwein W, Strasser T, Loeschke K (1989) Supplementation with *n*-3 fatty acids from fish oil in chronic inflammatory bowel disease – a randomised, placebo-controlled, double-blind cross-over trial. *J Int Med* 225: 225–232

12 Best WR, Becktel JM, Singleton JW, Kern F (1976) Development of a Crohn's disease activity index (CDAI). *Gastroenterology* 70: 439–444

13 MatË J, Castanos J, Garcia-Samaniego, Pajares JM (1993) Does dietary fish oil maintain the remission of Crohn's disease (CD): a study case control. *Gastroenterol* 100: A–228

14 Lorenz-Meyer H, Bauer P, Nicolay C, Scheurlen C, Scheurlen M, Fleig WB, Maschler C

Schulz B, Carr L (1996) Omega-3 fatty acids and carbohydrate diet for maintenance of remission in Crohnís disease. *Scan J Gastroenterol* 31: 778–785

15 Brignola C, De Simone G, Belloli C, Iannone P, Belluzzi A, Gionchetti P, Campieri M, Barbara L (1994) Steroid treatment in active Crohn's disease: a comparison between two regimens of different duration. *Aliment Pharmacol Ther* 8: 465–468

16 Budiarso IT (1990) Fish oil versus olive oil. *Lancet* 336: 1313–1314

17 Petroni A, Blasevich M, Salami M, Papini N, Montedoro GF and Galli C (1995) Inhibition of platelet aggregation and eicosanoid production by phenolic components of olive oil. *Thromb Res* 78: 151–160

18 Petroni A, Blasevich M, Papini N, Salami M, Sala A, Galli C (1997) Inhibition of leukocyte leukotriene B4 production by an olive oil-derived phenol identified by mass-spectrometry. *Thromb Res* 87(3): 315–322

19 Appel LJ, Miller ER, Seidler AJ, Whelton PK (1993) Does supplementation of diet with "fish oil" reduce blood pressure? A meta-analysis of controlled following coronary angioplasty. *Arch Intern Med* 153: 1429–1438

20 O'Connors GT, Malenka DJ, Olmstead EM, Johnson PS, Hennekens CH (1992) A meta-analysis of randomised trials of fish oil in prevention of restenosis following coronary angioplasty. *Am J Prev Med* 8: 186–192

21 Kunzel U, Bertsch S (1990) Klinsche Erfahrungen mit einem standardiserten Fischölkonzentrat. Feldstudie mit 3958 hyperlipamischen Patienten in der Praxis des niedergelassenen Arztes. *Fortschr Med* 108: 437–442

22 El Boustani S, Colette C, Monnier L, Descomps B, Crastes de Paulet A, Mendy F (1987) Enteral Absorption in man of eicosapentaenoic acid in different chemical forms. *Lipids* 22: 711–714

23 Lawson LD,Hughes BG (1988) Human absorption of fish oil fatty acids as triacylglycerols, free acids, or ethyl esters. *Bioch Bioph Res Comm* 152: 328–335

24 Belluzzi A, Brignola C, Campieri M, Camporesi E, Gionchetti P, Rizzello F, Belloli C, De Simone G, Boschi S, Miglioli M et al (1994) Effects of a new fish oil derivative on fatty acid phospholipid-membrane pattern in a group of Crohn's disease patients. *Dig Dis Sci* 39: 2589–2594

25 Wright JP, Alp MN, Young GD, Tigler Wibrandi N (1987) Predictors of acute relapse of Crohn's Disease: a laboratory and clinical study. *Dig Dis Sci* 32: 164–170

26 Brignola C, Campieri M, Bazzocchi G, Farruggia P, Tragnone A , Lanfranchi GA (1986) A laboratory index for predicting relapse in asymptomatic patients with Crohn's disease. *Gastroenterology* 91: 1490–1494.

27 Gendre JP, Mary JY, Modigliani R, Colombel JF, Soulé JC, Galmiche JP, Lerebours E, Descos L, Viteau JM, René E et al (1993) Oral mesalamine (Pentasa) maintenance treatment in Crohn's disease: a multicenter placebo-controlled study. *Gastroenterology* 104: 435–439

28 Belluzzi A, Brignola C, Campieri M, Pera A, Boschi S and Miglioli M (1996) Effect of an enteric-coated fish oil preparation on relapses in Crohn's disease. *New Engl J Med* 334: 1557–1616

29 Belluzzi A, Brignola C, Campieri M, Belloli C, Boschi S, Cottone M, Rizzello F, Miglioli M (1997) A new enteric coated preparation of omega 3 fatty acids for preventing post-surgical recurrence in Crohn's disease. Abstract book – Digestive Disease Week – Washington May 1997
30 Williams JG, Wong WD, Rothenberger DA, Goldberg SM (1991) Recurrence of Crohn's disease after resection. *Br J Surg* 78: 10–19
31 Basilisco G, Campanini M, Cesana B, Ranzi T, Bianchi P (1989). Risk factors for first operation in Crohn's disease. *Am J Gastroenterol* 84: 749–752
32 Olaison G, Smedh K, Sjodahl R (1992) Natural course of Crohn's disease after ileocolic resection: endoscopically visualised ileal ulcers preceding symptoms. *Gut* 33: 331–335.
33 Rutgeers P, Geboes K, Vantrappen G, Beyls J, Kerremans R, Hiele M (1990) Predictability of the postoperative course of Crohn's disease. *Gastroenterology* 99: 956–963
34 Shoda R, Matsueda K, Yamato S, Umeda N (1996) Epidemiologic analysis of Crohn disease in Japan: increased dietary intake of *n*-6 polyunsaturated fatty acids and animal protein relates to the increased incidence of Crohn disease in Japan. *Am J Clin Nutr* 63(5): 741–745

n-3 Fatty acids in the treatment of ulcerative colitis

John B. Rodgers

Albany Medical College, Department of Medicine, 47 New Scotland Ave., Albany, NY 12208, USA

Overview

Ulcerative colitis is a chronic inflammatory disease of the large bowel of unknown etiology. The inflammation is generally confined to the mucosal layers, resulting in extensive superficial ulceration. Antiinflammatory drugs are helpful in treating this condition, as are drugs that reduce the immune response such as azathioprine and 6-mercaptopurine. Fish oil *n*-3 polyunsaturated fatty acids (PUFAs), eicosapentaenoic (EPA) and docosahexaenoic acids (DHA), alter the production of leukotrienes by the lipoxygenase pathway and prostaglandins via the cyclooxygenase pathway. The major fatty acid for leukotriene synthesis is arachidonic acid (AA), which is the substrate for leukotriene B_4 (LTB_4). This cytokine is formed primarily by inflammatory cells [1] and its main role in the inflammatory reaction appears to be recruitment of neutrophils from the circulation to the inflamed tissue. When EPA is the substrate for this pathway, however, the product is leukotriene B_5 (LTB_5) which has only 10% of the activity of LTB_4 with regards to inducing neutrophil aggregation [2]. Furthermore, when AA and EPA are incubated together the production of LTB_4 is reduced by 68% [2]. In humans consuming a diet supplemented with fish oil, the 5-lipoxygenase pathway in both neutrophils and monocytes was reduced, and the adherence of neutrophils to vessel endothelium was inhibited completely. Additionally these neutrophils displayed less chemotactic response to LTB_4 [3].

The rationale for the use of fish oil to treat inflammatory bowel disease is strengthened by studies in patients suffering from this condition. The colonic mucosa from these patients contained more LTB_4 and synthesized more of this cytokine than the mucosa from normal subjects [4]. Additionally, in patients with ulcerative colitis involving the rectum, a significant reduction of LTB_4 and prostaglandin E_2 was observed in rectal dialysates after treatment with topical prednisolone, as compared to values prior to treatment [5]. These observations suggest that cytokines synthesized in the diseased colon are involved in the development of the inflammatory process and that successful treatment of the condition is the result, at least in part, of a reduction in LTB_4 synthesis in the colon.

Medicinal Fatty Acids in Inflammation, edited by J.M. Kremer

Dietary lipids have been shown to be incorporated into colonic mucosal lipids. Patients with inflammatory bowel disease given dietary fish oil had an increased recovery of EPA and DHA in colonic biopsy samples, and a reduced synthesis of prostaglandin E_2 and thromboxane B_2 [6]. Synthesis of LTB_4 was not assayed. However, others [7] have subsequently shown that recoveries of LTB_4 in the colonic lumen of patients with ulcerative colitis were lowered with fish oil treatment. Eleven patients given fish oil appeared to improve, based on the observation that the requirement for prednisolone was reduced as determined in follow up visits [6]. Considering these observations, plus the results of other studies documenting increased production of LTB_4 in diseased colonic tissue [4] and the decreased production of this cytokine by the colon in response to antiinfammatory medication [5], it would be reasonable to expect that treatment of ulcerative colitis patients with fish oil would be beneficial possibly as a result of decreasing the production of LTB_4 in the colon.

Fish oil has a number of effects on the immune system and it is possible that other factors other than decreased production of LTB_4 are involved in any benefit this agent might have. In this regard it was observed by Hiller et al. [6] that patients with inflammatory bowel disease treated with either fish oil or olive oil tended to improve, judged by the observation that the dose of prednisolone could be decreased, regardless which dietary oil the patients had been given. Olive oil had no effect on colonic mucosal eicosanoid synthesis and yet patients appeared to respond to this treatment.

Other cytokines are affected by fish oil. In humans the production of interleukin-1 and tumor necrosis factor was reduced by peripheral blood mononuclear cells after treatment for six weeks [8]. PUFAs have also been shown to suppress lymphocyte proliferation in humans [9, 10]. In a detailed study in the rat, analyzing the effects of different dietary lipids on various lymphocyte populations, it was observed that all fats including saturated fats (hydrogenated coconut oil) decreased proliferation of lymphocytes from the spleen but not from the thymus. Olive oil, evening primrose oil, and fish oil (menhaden oil) additionally inhibited proliferation of lymphocytes from mesenteric lymph nodes [11]. In these studies olive oil produced approximately the same results as fish oil. Additionally, the effect of *n*-3 PUFAs on the basic step of antigen-presenting cell function of human blood monocytes has been determined [12]. Both DHA and EPA were observed to decrease this process indicating that these fish oil fatty acids can influence the immune reactivity by modulating antigen-presenting cell function. The effects of other PUFAs were not investigated in this study.

As *n*-3 PUFAs have a variety of mechanisms to reduce the immune and inflammatory responses, it was appropriate to study the effects of fish oil in patients with ulcerative colitis. One of the first studies to address this question was reported by McCall et al. [13] who enrolled six patients and six healthy controls into an open label study, each receiving fish oil for a period of 12 weeks at a sufficient dose to supply 3–4 g of EPA daily. There was a significant improvement in patients' symptoms and histological appearance of the rectal mucosa at the termination of treatment. This was associated with a reduction of neutrophil LTB_4 levels. Also, the serum from patients was significantly less chemotactic for neutrophils compared to that observed for control serum.

In another preliminary report by Salomon et al. [14] ten patients with mild to moderate ulcerative colitis were given fish oil in an open label trial. Seven patients showed improvement and four of five patients on prednisolone were able to reduce the dose of this drug.

Following these preliminary reports four placebo controlled, double blind studies have been published describing results of fish oil treatment of patients with ulcerative colitis [7, 15–17]. Two studies [7, 15] reported positive findings for this treatment whereas the other two studies [16, 17] were less enthuthiastic. The latter two studies enrolled many patients who were in remission at the start of the treatment period. A single treatment, either an active agent or the placebo, was continued throughout the entire study lasting six [17] or twelve [16] months. The former two [7,15] were crossover studies with a one or two month washout period between treatment periods. In all four studies, antiinflammatory drugs being taken by any of the patients were continued, with attempts to reduce or discontinue these drugs as the studies progressed.

A report indicating clear benefit for fish oil treatment was that of Stenson et al. [7]. This was a multicenter, crossover trial with two treatment periods of four months, each with a one month washout period between the two treatment periods. Patients were randomized to receive 18 capsules of fish oil per day containing 3.24 g of EPA and 2.16 g of DHA, or 18 capsules containing isocaloric amounts of vegetable oil for the first treatment period. After the washout period, the other dietary oil supplement was given. Patients were evaluated at the end of each treatment program with a standard history and physical examination, a flexible sigmoidoscopy plus biopsy, and a rectal dialysate to measure prostaglandin E_2 and LTB_4. The gross and microscopic appearance of the sigmoid colon was evaluated using a standard scoring system. Twenty-four patients with active ulcerative colitis with diarrhea and rectal inflammation were enrolled, and eighteen finished the protocol and were evaluated.

Patients themselves could not discern any improvement in how they felt overall during one treatment period as compared to the other. However, the levels of LTB4 in the rectal dialysates were significantly reduced with fish oil treatment, and the histologic scores for the pathologic abnormalities of the sigmoid colon were significantly improved. There was also a trend for improvement of the scores in the gross appearance of the sigmoid colon. During the fish oil period, the patient gained a significant amount of weight, which was not observed after treatment with placebo. Finally, the dose of prednisolone in the seven patients taking fish oil was decreased from an average of 12.9 mg/day to 6.1 mg/day, while no reduction was possible on placebo. Thus, while there was no subjective data to indicate benefit for fish oil treatment, various objective measurements made during the study did indicate that fish oil treatment was of benefit for this condition.

In another study showing positive results for fish oil, Aslan and coworkers [15] enrolled eleven patients with mild to moderate ulcerative colitis into a crossover study where patients received enough fish oil daily to supply 4.2 g/day of *n*-3 fatty acids for three months, or placebo supplying an isocaloric amount of corn oil for the first treatment period. After a two month washout period, the other treatment was given. The patients were evaluated by changes in the disease activity index as determined at the beginning and end of each treatment period. The mean disease activity index declined 56% by the end of the fish oil period and declined only 4% after placebo treatment. This difference was statistically significant. In addition, the dose of antiinflammatory drugs was reduced in eight of eleven patients while on fish oil. Patients were also evaluated by determining scores of histologic abnormalities of rectal biopsies obtained at the end of each treatment period and by measuring mucosal LTB4 production. No differences were observed for these two sets of data. The authors concluded that fish oil produces clinical improvement in patients with mild to moderate ulcerative colitis.

In another randomized, placebo controlled study [16] eighty seven patients with ulcerative colitis were enrolled and given liquid fish oil daily to supply 4.5 g/day of EPA or olive oil as the placebo. Treatment was continued for one year. Forty five patients were given fish oil and forty two patients received placebo. 42% of patients assigned to fish oil and 36% of patients assigned to placebo were in remission at the start of treatment, and another 36% and 45% respectively achieved remission during treatment that lasted at least four weeks. However, maintenance of remission was not enhanced by fish oil in 54% of patients in the fish oil group, and 63% of patients in the placebo group noted to relapse by the end of one year of treatment. The only possible benefit noted was for patients with active disease at entry into the study. For these patients given fish oil there was a significant reduction in corticosteroid requirement after several months of treatment. Additionally there was a tendency for patients with active disease to achieve remission off corticosteroids faster if given fish oil, but results were not statistically significant when compared to those of patients treated with placebo. Thus the only benefit these investigators observed with fish oil was a corticosteroid sparing effect in patients with active disease.

In the last of the four publications analyzing the possible benefits of fish oil in the treatment of ulcerative colitis [17] three groups of patients with stable disease were randomized to receive either fish oil, super evening primrose oil, or placebo (olive oil) for six months. For the purposes of this review only the results for fish oil will be described. The dose of fish oil was relatively small, 12 capsules of 1 g daily for one month followed by 6 capsules daily for the next five months. Therefore, for most of the study period patients on fish oil received 1.1 g of EPA and 0.73 g of DHA daily. Except for one patient with moderate disease, patients enrolled had mild disease or were in remission. Only two were taking corticosteroids at the time of entry into the study. Outcome of treatment was assessed by patient diary cards, sigmoidoscopy and histology of rectal biopsy specimens. On analysis of the data no benefit was identified for fish oil.

What are we to conclude from these studies regarding possible benefits of fish oil in patients with ulcerative colitis? First, it appears that benefit is more likely if the dose of fish oil is relatively high. Thus, in the study describing the greatest benefit [7] patients received 5.4 g of *n*-3 PUFAs daily, whereas in the study reporting no benefit [17] the daily dose was only 1.8 g. Second, fish oil at high doses is beneficial but the effects are very subtle and are not appreciated by the patients themselves. This fact, plus the requirement to take multiple fish oil tablets daily for prolonged periods of time, would likely affect patient compliance. If patients do not obviously feel better on any given agent they are not likely to take the agent as instructed especially if it has unpleasant side effects as fish oil does. Third, it appears that benefit for fish oil is easier to demonstrate if patients with mild to moderate disease are studied as opposed to evaluating possible benefits of fish oil in patients in remission. Three of the studies [7, 15, 16] demonstrated that when fish oil was given to patients with moderate disease the dose of corticosteroids could be lowered. In the one study that did not verify this observation [17] only two patients were on corticosteroids on enrollment.

The fact that fish oil treatment did not keep patients in remission any longer than the placebo (olive oil) did is troubling [17]. This is surprising since fish oil was recently reported to maintain remission in patients with Crohn's disease [18]. The formulation of the fish oil was quite different in the study of Crohn's patients, making the agent less objectionable thus tending to improve patient compliance. The other difference in the design of this study was the choice of the placebo which was a combination of caprylic and capric acids presented in the triglyceride form. These are medium chain fats which, following absorption, would likely be rapidly oxidized or used as substrate to make saturated fats such as palmitate. This placebo, therefore, would not be expected to have much effect on the immune mechanism as has been described above for olive oil and certain *n*-6 PUFAs. Olive oil and corn oil, used as the placebo for the studies of patients with ulcerative colitis was likely not the best choice. Although treatment with olive or corn oil would not reduce the production of LTB_4, it is not clear that the benefits of fish oil in these patients is mainly the result of reducing the levels of this cytokine in the colon. *n*-3 PUFAs and other unsaturated long chain fatty acids have a number of effects on the immune mechanism, as mentioned, so that a comparison of possible benefit between fish oil and other dietary oils containing mainly long chain unsaturated fats might be expected to show little difference, especially when the patients are not ill but in remission. In this regard, in one of the preliminary studies in patients with inflammatory bowel disease [6] the results noted with placebo treatment (olive oil) were comparable to those observed for fish oil. It would certainly be of interest to repeat studies of fish oil in patients with ulcerative colitis using a high dose given in the formulation used in the Crohn's study [18] comparing the results with those obtained with a placebo that has no modulating effect on the immune mechanism.

References

1 Lee TH, Austen F (1985) Arachidonic acid metabolism by the 5-lipoxygenase pathway, and the effects of alternative dietary fatty acids. *Adv Immunol* 39: 145–175

2 Prescott SM (1984) The effect of eicosapentaenoic acid of leukotriene B production by human neutrophils. *J Biol Chem* 259: 7615–7621

3 Lee TH, Hoover RL, Williams JD, Sperling RI, Ravalese J, Spur BW, Robinson DR, Corey EJ, Lewis RA, Austen KF (1985) Effect of dietary enrichment with eicosapentaenoic and docosahexaenoic acids on *in vitro* neutrophil and monocyte leukotriene generation and neutrophil function. *N Engl J Med* 312: 1217–1224

4 Sharon P, Stenson WF (1984) Enhanced synthesis of leukotriene B_4 by colonic mucosa in inflammatory bowel disease. *Gastroenterology* 86: 453–460

5 Lauritsen K, Laursen LS, Bukhave K, Rask-Madsen J (1986) Effect of topical 5-aminosalicylic acid and prednisolone on prostaglandin E_2 and leukotriene B_4 levels determined by equilibrium *in vitro* dialysis of rectum in relapsing ulcerative colitis. *Gastroenterology* 91: 837–844

6 Hiller K, Jewell R, Dorrell L, Smith CL (1991) Incorporation of fatty acids from fish oil and olive oil into colonic mucosal lipids and effects upon eicosanoid synthesis in inflammatory bowel disease. *Gut* 32: 1151–1155

7 Stenson WF, Cort D, Rodgers J, Burakoff R, DeSchryver-Kecskemetti K, Gramlich TL, Beeken W (1992) Dietary supplementation with fish oil in ulcerative colitis. *Ann Intern Med* 116: 609–614

8 Enders S, Ghorbani R, Kelley VE, Georgilis K, Lonnemann G, van der Meer JWM, Cannon JG, Rogers TS, Klempner MS, Weber PC et al (1989) The effect of dietary supplementation with *n*-3 polyunsaturated fatty acids on the synthesis of interleukin-1 and tumor necrosis factor by mononuclear cells. *N Engl J Med* 320: 265–271

9 Calder PC, Newsholme EA (1992) Polyunsaturated fatty acids suppress human peripheral blood lymphocyte proliferation and interleukin-2 production. *Clin Sci* 82: 695–700

10 Meydani SN, Endres S, Woods MM, Goldin BR, Soo C, Morrill-Labrode A, Dinarello C, Gorbach SL (1991) Oral (*n*-3) fatty acid supplementation suppresses cytokine production and lymphocyte proliferation: comparison between young and older women. *J Nutr* 121: 547–555

11 Yaqoob P, Newsholme EA, Calder PC (1994) The effect of dietary lipid manipulation on rat lymphocyte subsets and proliferation. *Immunology* 82: 603–610

12 Hughes DA, Southon S, Pinder AC (1996) (*n*-3) Polyunsaturated fatty acids modulate the expression of functionally associated molecules on human monocytes *in vitro*. *J Nutr* 126: 603–610

13 McCall TB, O'Leary D, Bloomfield J, O'Morain CA (1989) Therapeutic potential of fish oil in the treatment of ulcerative colitis. *Aliment Pharmacol Ther* 3: 415–424
14 Salomon P, Kornbluth AA, Janowitz HD (1990) Treatment of ulcerative colitis with fish oil *n*-3-w-fatty acid: an open trial. *J Clin Gastroenterol* 12: 157–161
15 Aslan A, Triadafilopoulos G (1992) Fish oil fatty acid supplementation in active ulcerative colitis: a double-blind, placebo-controlled, crossover study. *Amer J Gastroenterol* 87: 432–437
16 Hawthorne AB, Daneshmend TK, Hawkey CJ, Belluzzi A, Everitt SJ, Holmes GKT, Malkinson C, Shaheen MZ, Willars JE (1992) Treatment of ulcerative colitis with fish oil supplementation: a prospective 12 month randomized controlled trial. *Gut* 33: 922–928
17 Greenfield SM, Green AT, Teare JP, Jenkins AP, Punchard NA, Ainley CC, Thompson RPH (1993) A randomized controlled study of evening primrose and fish oil in ulcerative colitis. *Aliment Pharmacol Ther* 7: 159–166
18 Belluzzi A, Brignola C, Campieri M, Pera A, Boschi S, Miglioli M (1996) Effect of an enteric-coated fish-oil preparation on relapses in Crohn's disease. *N Engl J Med* 334: 1557–1560

13. McCall TB, O'Leary D, Bloomfield J, O'Morain CA (1989) Therapeutic potential of fish oil in the treatment of ulcerative colitis. Aliment Pharmacol Ther 3: 415-424
14. Salomon P, Kornbluth AA, Janowitz HD (1990) Treatment of ulcerative colitis with fish oil n-3-ω-fatty acid: an open trial. J Clin Gastroenterol 12: 157-161
15. Aslan A, Triadafilopoulos G (1992) Fish oil fatty acid supplementation in active ulcerative colitis: a double-blind, placebo-controlled, crossover study. Am J Gastroenterol 87: 432-437
16. Hawthorne AB, Daneshmend TK, Hawkey CJ, Belluzzi A, Everitt SJ, Holmes GKT, Malkinson C, Shaheen MZ, Willars JE (1992) Treatment of ulcerative colitis with fish oil supplementation: a prospective 12 month randomised controlled trial. Gut 33: 922-928
17. Greenfield SM, Green AT, Teare JP, Jenkins AP, Punchard NA, Ainley CC, Thompson RPH (1993) A randomized controlled study of evening primrose oil and fish oil in ulcerative colitis. [illegible]
18. [illegible]

n-3 Fatty acids in the treatment of rheumatoid arthritis

Piet P. Geusens

Clinical Research Center for Bone and Joint Diseases, Dr. L. Willems-Instituut, Limburgs Universitair Centrum, B-3590 Diepenbeek, Belgium

Summary. The pathophysiology of rheumatoid arthritis (RA) is complex and still not fully understood. Currently the main hypothesis is that chronic inflammation occurs after stimulation by T cell-macrophage interaction, induced by unknown antigen(s). This is accompanied by a complex sequence of highly integrated actions between macrophages, synoviocytes, polymorphonuclear cells and endothelial cells. The chronic inflammation is a major cause of pain and functional impairment, ultimately resulting in joint destruction. The production of eicosanoids (prostaglandins and leukotrienes) by macrophages/synoviocytes is only one of the many pathways of the inflammatory reaction, but the well-established efficacy of NSAIDs in patients with RA underscores the importance of the pro-inflammatory cyclo-oxygenase-pathway products in the pathophysiology of the symptoms. A positive clinical effect of *n*-3 fatty acids has been shown in some but not all animal experiments of arthritis. In patients with RA, *n*-3 fatty acid supplementation decreased clinical symptoms. Differences from patients treated with placebo (but still on NSAIDs or disease modifying drugs) were significant in some studies. A significant difference from placebo in the tender joint score and morning stiffness was found in a meta- and mega-analysis of 10 studies. In long-term studies, treatment with *n*-3 fatty acids resulted in a substantial decrease of the use of NSAIDs and/or disease modifying drugs as compared to placebo. No effects have been documented on the progression of joint destruction. No major side effects were reported compared to placebo. Therefore, as part of the total treatment program of RA, patients should be advised about the potential moderate effects on their symptoms of diet supplements with *n*-3 fatty acids.

Introduction

Rheumatoid arthritis (RA) is a systemic illness with chronic, symmetric polyarthritis as its most important clinical feature. RA usually starts with inflammation in the joints with swelling, pain, functional impairment, morning stiffness, disuse osteoporosis and muscle wasting. Typical for RA is the development of erosions, which develop in approximately 70–75% of the patients in the hand and feet. Subcutaneous nodules occur often in progressive disease. Extra-articular manifestations, such as pericarditis, pleuritis, Felty's syndrome, and vasculitis exist in a minority of the patients. Features include presence of rheumatoid factors in the serum in most patients with severe disease, elevated acute phase proteins, and secondary anaemia.

The aetiology of RA is still unknown, and seems to be multifactorial. The currently most frequent studied hypothesis is that a (still unknown) antigen activates the immune system by presentation by an antigen presenting cell to T cells in a

Medicinal Fatty Acids in Inflammation, edited by J.M. Kremer

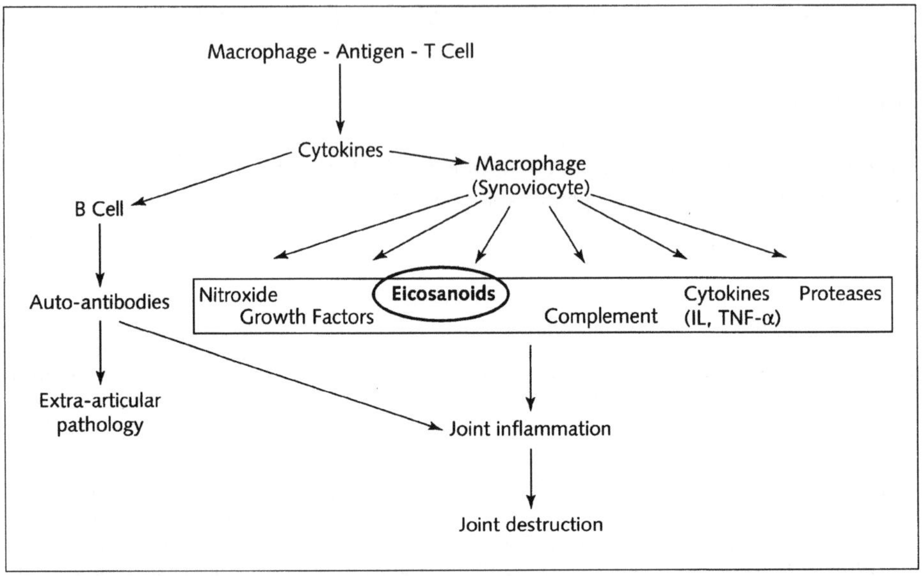

Figure 1
Pathophysiology of rheumatoid arthritis according to the hypothesis of causative (auto)antigen(s). IL denotes interleukin; TNF-α denotes tumor necrosis factor.

genetically predisposed subject involving human leukocyte antigen (HLA)-DR4 [1] (Fig. 1). Subsequently chronic inflammation develops, due to persistence of the antigen stimulus or the appearance of new antigens (e.g. released during tissue destruction). T cells, macrophages, polymorphonuclear cells and synovial fibroblast-like cells (synoviocytes) are involved. The chronic inflammation is characterised by a heterogeneous inflammatory cell population that produce eicosanoids, cytokines, growth factors and enzymes, resulting in hypertrophied synovitis and the pannus, and in systemic changes such as the production of rheumatoid factors and immune complexes, that can cause vasculitis. The destruction of the joints is related to the appearance of the pannus, a unique histologic feature of RA [2].

Not only is the aetiology unknown, no curative treatment of RA is known either [3]. The major aims in the treatment of RA are alleviation of the signs and symptoms of active inflammation, prevention of tissue destruction, preservation of function and reversal of phenomena threatening organ function. Important aspects of the treatment of RA include patient education, counselling, physical therapy, pharmacotherapy, surgery and occupational therapy. Pharmacotherapy, still the mainstay of the treatment of RA, is divided into first- and second-line drugs. First-line drugs such as non-steroidal anti-inflammatory drugs (NSAIDs) give immediate relief of pain and stiffness. They inhibit the joint inflammation, but do not influence the natural course of the disease. The second-line drugs are called disease-modifying anti-rheumatic drugs (DMARDs) and are characterised by the capacity to alter the course of the disease. Most second-line drugs have a delayed onset of action and do not interfere directly with the metabolism of eicosanoids. Corticosteroids are an exception and are potent anti-inflammatory drugs used orally or intra-articularly in the treatment of RA. They have a broad spectrum of actions one of which is their influence on the metabolism of eicosanoids. They inhibit the activity of phospholipase A_2 by the release of an inhibitory protein, lipocortin+1^{34}, that has the ability to bind calcium and anionic phospholipids (for review see [4]). Corticosteroids also inhibit the expression of cyclo-oxygenase II (COX-2) [5].

Current pharmacological treatment of RA still suffers from problems with compliance and toxicity in a high percentage of patients. As an example, most DMARDs (with the exception of methotrexate) are stopped after one year due to side effects [6]. Furthermore, the potential toxicity of NSAIDs on gastric mucosa and renal function has led to the extensive research for the value of COX-2 selective inhibitors [7]. Furthermore, in spite of positive effects on disease progression in clinical trials, long-term observations indicate that the RA is still progressive [8].

Diet manipulation had until recently not the interest in RA as in other diseases such as cardiovascular diseases or diabetes. As several double-blind controlled studies with favourable effect have been published [9–20], we will in this overview concentrate on the rationale and the effects of *n*-3 fatty acid supplementation in patients with RA.

Eicosanoid metabolism in animal models of auto-immune disease

In animal models of arthritis, increased COX-2 expression and activity was found in joint tissues of rats [21] and in other animal models of acute and chronic inflammation [22, 23].

Alterations after *n*-3 fatty acids supplements in animal models of inflammation

Dietary manipulation of *n*-3 fatty acids reduces the severity of glomerulonephritis in several auto-immune strains of mice (NZBxNZWF1, BxSB/Mpj and MRL/lpr) [24–28], even when added after the start of the disease [24]. However, not all studies on *n*-3 fatty acid manipulation in animal models showed favourable effects. In the type II collagen arthritis model in rats the incidence of arthritis increased [25] and in systemic lupus erythematosus (SLE) in MRL/lpr mice the incidence of vasculitis was increased [25].

Eicosanoid metabolism in RA

The biochemical alterations after *n*-3 fatty acids supplements in patients with RA have been reviewed in detail (see Fernandes, this volume, and [29–33]). In summary, COX-1 and COX-2 expression are increased in synovium of RA patients [21]. Synoviocytes are the major source of prostaglandins (PGs) in synovial tissue of RA [5]. In synovial fluid of patients with active RA several inflammatory active metabolites of eicosanoids were found in biologically significant concentrations, such as PGE_2, leukotriene-B_4 (LTB_4), 5-hydroperoxyeicosatetraenoic acid (5-HETE) and platelet-activating factor (PAF) [29]. An increase in LTB_4 has also been documented in patients with juvenile RA [34]. These metabolites have multiple actions in synovial inflammation. PGE_2 is pro-inflammatory in that it enhances the chemotactic activity and vasodilative properties of LTB_4, complement-5a, histamine and kinines [29]. PGE_2 enhances the evocation of pain, induces (local) pyrexia, increases blood flow and stimulates osteoclastic bone resorption, that results in the early radiological changes of peri-articular osteoporosis in RA [29, 35]. LTB_4 increases vascular permeability, enhances local blood flow, is one of the most potent chemotaxins and inhibits lymphocyte activation and proliferation [29]. 5-HETE is an agonist for the LTB_4 receptor [29]. PAF can stimulate tumor necrosis factor (TNF) as well as other cytokines in endothelial tissue and is 1000 times more potent than histamine in inducing changes in vascular permeability [29]. Evidence suggests that PAF also can modulate T cell and monocyte function [32].

It is clear that the acutely increased production of PG plays a critical role in acute inflammatory processes [7]. The role of PG in the development and maintenance of chronic inflammation is far more complex. Pro-inflammatory cytokines increase PG production in synoviocytes [5] and interleukin-1 (IL-1) increases PG production in macrophages, endothelial cells, osteoblasts and chondrocytes [36]. The *in vivo* effects of increased COX expression are likely to be pleiotropic [7]. As an example, inhibition of COX exacerbates cartilage erosion, but reduces bone loss [7]. PG production has been implicated in the production of matrix metalloproteinases expression by synoviocytes [37], and in angiogenesis [36].

Biochemical alterations after *n*-3 fatty acids supplements in patients with RA

In several studies in patients with RA the biochemical effects of *n*-3 fatty acids have been documented (for reviews see [29–33]). Eicosapentaeoic acid (EPA) inhibited the formation of LTB_4 by activated neutrophils and monocytes [11]. LTB_5, derived from EPA, possesses only 10% of the bioactivity of LTB_4 and also partially inhibits LTB_4 [29]. EPA may suppress PAF formation by monocytes [32] and suppressed production of IL-1 and IL-1β [20, 39] but no changes were found in IL-2, IL-6 and IL-8 [20]. No inhibition on TNF-α production could be demonstrated in RA [20] as was documented in healthy volunteers [40]. After fish oil diet, there was a normalisation of the depressed neutrophile function [38]. This unexpected finding is not already well explained and could be related to the experimental environment or the concomitant use of NSAIDs [29]. No effects on acute phase proteins could be shown.

Some other effects of EPA that could be of potential clinical interest have been documented in healthy volunteers or *in vitro* – but until now not in patients with RA – such as inhibition of TNF-α production [40], the suppression of production of metalloproteinase expression in synoviocytes [37], inhibition of angiogenesis [36] and modulation of intracellular signal transduction involved in cell proliferation and differentiation [41, 42].

Clinical results of *n*-3 fatty acids supplements in patients with RA

Some evidence for clinical importance of *n*-3 fatty acids in diet comes from cross-sectional data. When comparing dietary intake of fatty acids in 324 women with RA to 1245 healthy women, a decreased risk for RA was reported with consumption of broiled or baked fish, but not of other types of fish [43]. The odds ratio (OR) for the use of ≥ 2 servings of broiled or baked fish per week (compared to < 1 serving) was 0.57 (95% confidence interval (CI) = 0.35 to 0.93). Furthermore, patients with RA have several dietary deficiencies compared to the Recommended Dietary Allowance (RDA), including insufficient poly-unsaturated fatty acids [44].

Most convincing results of EPA come from prospective studies in RA. *n*-3 fatty acid supplementation has been studied in at least 12 prospective double-blind placebo-controlled studies with different design and duration (Tab. 1) [9–20]. These studies were performed in patients with long-standing RA (mean duration from 8 to 15 years) with a mean age between 50 and 61 years. Mean intake of *n*-3 fatty acids (fish oil + EPA + docosaheaenoic acid (DHA)) varied from 1.0 to 7.1 g/day (median: 3.3 g).

In 11 of the studies in which clinical parameters were measured, an improvement compared to baseline in at least two clinical parameters was found after supplementation with *n*-3 fatty acids. A decrease in the number of tender joints (an average of 31%) was the most consistent finding, together with amelioration of several other clinical parameters according to the study (Tab. 1). As the aim of double-blind studies is to compare the effect versus the control group, we will discuss these comparisons in more detail. Although in all studies placebo was used, no study involved a real placebo. First, all placebo treated patients used a heterogeneous group of dietary control oils. Vegetable oils cannot be taken as true placebo as clinical effects have been suggested [32]. Second, in most studies patients continued NSAIDs or DMARDs in the treatment and in the placebo group. In studies on the effect of NSAIDs, the use of other NSAIDs was generally an exclusion criterion [33] and in

Table 1 - Summary of the double-blind clinical studies of n-3 fatty acid supplementation in patients with RA

Study [reference]	n	Duration of study (months)	Concomitant medication	*n*-3 fatty acid supplement (g/day) EPA*	DHA**	Outcome measurements which improved after fish oil: compared to baseline	compared to placebo
Kremer [9]	37	3	continued	1.8	1.2	morning stiffness, tender joints	
Kremer [10]	33	3.5	continued	2.7	1.8	ARA class, physician's global time to fatigue, tender joints swollen joints	time to fatigue, tender joints
Cleland [11]	46	3	continued	3.2	2.0	tender joints, grip strength	
Kremer [12]	49	6	continued (change was withdrawal criterion)	low: 1.7 high: 3.5	1.2# 2.4	swollen joints, tender joints, grip strength, morning stiffness, physician's global (high dose only)	grip strength, n of clinical clinical measures that ameliorated
Tulliken [13]	27	3	continued	2.0	1.3	swollen joints, joint pain index	joint pain index, Ritchie index, swollen joints
van der Tempel [14]	16	3	continued	2.0	1.3	swollen joints, morning stiffness	
Skoldham [15]	43	6	continued DMARD, free to change NSAID	1.8	1.2	physician's global, Ritchie index, decreased NSAID use	
Kjeldsen-Kragh [16]	67	4	NSAID continued in group A and stopped at 10 weeks in group B	3.8	2.0	Ritchie index, morning stiffness	morning stiffness

Table 1 (continued)

Study [reference]	n	Duration of study (months)	Concomitant medication	*n*-3 fatty acid supplement (g/day) EPA*	DHA**	Outcome measurements which improved after fish oil: compared to baseline	compared to placebo
Nielsen [17]	51	3	continued	2.0	1.2	morning stiffness, tender joints, CRP	morning stiffness, tender joints, patient pain
Lau [18]	64	12+3	no DMARD, change in NSAID was endpoint	1.7	1.1	decreased NSAID use	
Geusens [19]	60	12	varied as required during the study	low: 0.8 high: 1.7	0.2 0.4	patient global, physician pain, decreased NSAID and/or DMARD (high dose only)	patient global, physician pain, decreased NSAID and/or DMARD (high dose only)
Kremer [20]	49	6 to 7	continued DMARD and NSAID, but NSAID stopped at 18 or 22 weeks	4.6	2.5#	tender joints, morning stiffness, physician pain, patient global (at 18 or 22 weeks)	DMARD (high dose only), tender joints

**EPA = eicosapentaeoic acid, ** DHA = docosaheanoic acid, # based on 65 kg subjects* studies with DMARDs, NSAID therapy is generally continued but other DMARDs were generally not allowed [33]. In spite of these limitations, significant ameliorations compared to placebo were documented for time to fatigue [10], swollen joints [10, 20], morning stiffness [17], tender joints [17] and patient global assessment [19], but the results were heterogeneous between the different studies. Therefore, the results of a meta-analysis were welcomed [45]. Ten studies were combined in a meta-analysis (based on global results) and in a mega-analysis (based on the reanalysis of primary data) of 395 patients including patients of randomised, double-blind controlled studies treated for 3 months [28]. The significant improvement could be confirmed in tender joint count (rate difference (RD) (95% CI) = –2.9, –3.8 to –2.1, $p < 0.001$) and morning stiffness (RD = –25.9, –44.3 to –7.5, $p < 0.01$) as compared to heterogeneous dietary control oils. No other significant differences from placebo were found.

Two long-term studies lasting 1 year have been published [19, 46]. In the first long-term study the need for NSAIDs, which was the primary endpoint, was significantly decreased to 41% of the original dose [46]. In a second one-year study, (2.6 g/day) resulted in a significant amelioration compared to the baseline in physician's and patient's global assessment, physician's pain assessment and Ritchie articular index [19]. Patient's global assessment and the number of patients with overall improvement during the study significantly favoured fish oil supplements. The percentage of patients that could reduce the intake of NSAIDs and/or DMARDs was significant and was similar to the proportion of patients (±50%) reporting significant improvement in disease activity [19].

A reduction in indomethacin need was documented, but the result was not different from placebo [47]. Some studies indicate that a positive effect is maintained for some time after stopping EPA [20], as found *in vitro* [40]. There seemed to be a dose related effect as a more rapid amelioration was found if the dose of EPA was increased from 2.7 to 3.6 g/day [12]. Higher doses (> 9 g/day for a patient of 70 kg) were not more efficient and are not recommended [20]. The effect of EPA also seems related to the duration of its application [32].

The tolerance of EPA was similar to placebo, although no data are available about compliance at long-term (longer than 1 year). Gastric problems can be reduced by increasing the EPA dose gradually over a 2-week period [32].

The hypothesis that concurrent pharmacotherapy in RA could potentiate the effect of *n*-3 fatty acids or could lower the need for *n*-3 fatty acids [32] has not been addressed in a prospective study.

Supplementation with *n*-3 fatty acids was also studied in other auto-immune diseases. In patients with Crohn's disease in remission, enteric-coated fish oil (2.7 g/day) during 1 year was effective in reducing the rate of relapse (59% in the fish-oil group versus 26% in the placebo group, $p = 0.003$) [48]. This was accompanied by a significant reduction in biochemical serum-parameters of inflammation.

The effects of GLA in RA are discussed in the chapter by Zurier, this volume.

Dietary supplements with *n*-3 fatty acids of other sources than fish oil

Whether the high doses of *n*-3 fatty acids can be achieved by diet alone remains to be proven in terms of acceptability and compliance. Indeed, dietary supplements are difficult to achieve and demand extensive adaptation of current Western diets [33]. In order to suppress IL-1β and TNF-α, EPA levels should be increased to approximately 1% of total fatty acids [49] and a possible suppression of TNF-α still has to be proven in RA. Fish oils are the only concentrated source of EPA [50]. The major source of *n*-3 fatty acids in vegetables is α-linoleic acid (α-LNA). However, the use of α-LNA cannot be used as an alternative for EPA without caution on some fundamental differences between α-LNA and EPA [50]. α-LNA must be converted to EPA before it exerts biological effects similar to EPA. Humans convert α-LNA to EPA to a small extent and α-LNA may be more readily oxidised than incorporated into tissues. The effects of consuming α-LNA-rich oils are more modest than the effects of EPA. Further data on the use of α-LNA are therefore necessary in RA before advocating them as a substitute or additional source of *n*-3 fatty acids in the treatment of RA.

It should be stressed that other dietary factors could be important in RA and a global approach for dietary advice is indicated [33]. Furthermore, background diet containing high LA as in current Western diets could diminish the beneficial anti-inflammatory effects of dietary *n*-3 fatty acids and should therefore be avoided [33].

Recent data on treatment of RA in its early phase indicate that suppression of inflammation early after start of the disease could have long-term effect on disease progression but not on clinical parameters [51]. No data are available on the effects of *n*-3 fatty acid supplementation in early RA. As *n*-3 fatty acids do not lower acute phase proteins, they can only be an additive, but not an alternative for aggressive pharmacological treatment in active synovitis early in the disease.

Conclusions

Several studies indicate that *n*-3 fatty acids could be a valuable supportive therapy in patients with RA, and therefore dietary advice of *n*-3 fatty acid manipulation should be given to patients with RA. However, EPA administration is only one part of the total treatment program of RA as the ultimate goal of treatment is prevention of joint destruction and early suppression of inflammation. The preventive effect of relapses by *n*-3 fatty acids as reported in Crohn's disease, and the protective effect of *n*-3 fatty acid rich diet on the incidence of RA opens perspectives for further clinical studies in auto-immune diseases. There is a need for further well-designed double-blind controlled studies, involving appropriate controls as performed in recent drug studies, before definite conclusions on efficiency and tolerance in RA can be drawn.

References

1 Panayi GS, Lanchbury JS, Kingsley GH (1992) The importance of the T cell in initiating and maintaining the chronic synovitis of RA. *Arthritis Rheum* 35: 729–735
2 Harris ED (1989) Pathogenesis of RA. In: WN Kelley, ED Harris, S Ruddy, CB Sledge (eds): *Textbook of Rheumatology*. WB Saunders Company, 929–932
3 Pincus T, Callahan LF (1993) What is the natural history of rheumatoid Arthritis? *Rheumat Dis Clin N Amer* 19: 123–151
4 Flower RJ, Rothwell NJ (1994) Lipocortin-1: cellular mechanisms and clinical relevance. *Trends Pharmacol Sci* 15: 71–76
5 Crofford LJ, Wilder RL, Ristimaki SAP, Remmers EF, Epps HR, Hla T (1994) Cyclooxygenase-1 and -2 expression in rheumatoid synovial tissues: effect of interleukin-1β, phorbol ester, and corticosteroids. *J Clin Invest* 93: 1095–1101
6 Pincus T, Callahan LF (1993) Variability in individual responses of 532 patients with rheumatoid arthritis to first-line and second-line drugs. *Agents Actions Suppl* 44: 67–75
7 Vane J, Botting J, Botting R (eds) (1996) *Improved non-steroidal anti-inflammatory drugs: COX-2 enzyme inhibitors*. Kluwer Academic Publishers and William Harvey Press, Hingham, MA, USA
8 Pincus T (1992) The paradox of effective therapies but poor long-term outcome in rheumatoid arthritis. *Semin Arthritis Rheum* 21: 2–15
9 Kremer JM, Bigaouette J, Michalek AV, Timchalk MA, Lininger L, Rynes RI, Huyck C, Zieminski J, Bartholomew LE (1985) Effects of manipulation of dietary fatty acids on clinical manifestations of rheumatoid arthritis. *Lancet* 1: 184–187
10 Kremer JM, Jubiz W, Michalek A, Rynes RI, Bartholomew LE, Bigaouette J, Timchalk MA, Beeler D, Lininger L (1987) Fish-oil fatty acid supplementation in active rheumatoid arthritis. A double-blinded, controlled cross-over study. *Ann of Intern Med* 106: 497–502
11 Cleland LG, French JK, Betts WH, Murphy GA, Elliot MJ (1988) Clinical and biochemical effects of dietary fish oil supplements in rheumatoid arthritis. *J Rheumatol* 15: 1471–1475
12 Kremer JM, Lawrence DA, Jubiz W, DiGiacomo R, Rynes R, Bartholomew LE, Sherman M(1990) Dietary fish oil and olive oil supplementation in patients with rheumatoid arthritis. Clinical and immunologic effects. *Arthritis Rheum* 33: 810–820
13 Tulleken JE, Limburg PC, Muskiet FAJ, van Rijswijk MH (1990) Vitamin E status during dietary fish oil supplementation in rheumatoid arthritis. *Arthritis Rheum* 33: 1416–1419
14 Van der Tempel H, Tulleken JE, Limburg PC, Muskiet FAJ, van Rijswijk MH (1990) Effects of fish oil supplementation in rheumatoid arthritis. Ann Rheum Dis 49: 76–80
15 Skoldstam L, Borjesson O, Kjallman A, Seiving B, Akesson B (1992) Effect of six month of fish oil supplementation in stable rheumatoid arthritis: a double-blind, controlled study. *Scand J Rheumatol* 21: 178–185

16 Kjeldsen-Kragh J, Lund JA, Riise T, Finnanger B, Haaland K, Finstad R, Mikkelsen K, Forre O (1992) Dietary *n*-3 fatty acid supplementation and naproxen treatment in patients with rheumatoid arthritis. *J Rheum* 19: 1531–1536

17 Nielsen GL, Faarvang KL, Thomsen BS, Teglbjaerg KL, Jensen LT, Hansen TM, Lervang HH, Schmidt EB, Dyerberg J, Ernst E (1992) The effect of dietary supplementation with *n*-3 polyunsaturated fatty acids in patients with rheumatoid arthritis: a randomised, double blind trial. *Eur J Clin Invest* 22: 687–691

18 Lau CS, Morley KD, Belch JJF (1993) Effects of fish oil supplementation on non-steroidal anti-inflammatory drug requirement in patients with mild rheumatoid arthritis. *Br J Rheumatol* 32: 982–989

19 Geusens P, Wouters C, Nijs J, Jiang Y, Dequeker J (1994) Long-term effect of omega-3 fatty acid supplementation in active rheumatoid arthritis. *Arthritis Rheum* 37 (6), 824–829

20 Kremer JM, Lawrence DA, Petrillo GF, Litts LL, Mullaly PM, Rynes RL, Stocker RP, Parhami N, Greenstein NS, Fuchs BR, Mathur A, Robinson DR, Sperling RI, Bigaouette J (1995) The effect of high dose fish oil on rheumatoid arthritis after stopping NSAIDs: clinical and immune correlates in patients with rheumatoid arthritis. *Arthr Rheumat* 38: 1107–1114

21 Sano H, Hla T, Maier JAM et al (1992) *In vivo* cyclooxygenase expression in synovial tissues of patients with rheumatoid arthritis and osteoarthosis and rats with adjuvant and streptococcal cell wall arthritis. *J Clin Invest* 89: 97–108

22 Masferrer JL, Zweifel BS, Manning PT et al (1994) Selective inhibition of inducible cyclooxygenase 2 *in vivo* is antiinflammatory and nonulcerogenic. *Proc Natl Acad Sci USA* 91: 3228–3232

23 Vane JR, Mitchell JA, Appleton I et al (1994) Inducible isoforms of cyclooxygenase and nitric-oxide synthase in inflammation. *Proc Natl Acad Sci USA* 91: 2046–2050

24 Robinson DR, Prickett JD, Makoul GT, Steinber AD, Colvin RB (1986) Dietary fish oil reduces progression of established renal disease in (NZB x NZW) mice and delays renal disease in BXSB and MRL/1 strains. *Arthritis Rheum* 29: 539–546

25 Prickett JD, Trentham DE, Robinson DR (1984) Dietary fish oil augments the induction of arthritis in rats immunised with type II collagen. *J Immunol* 132: 725–729

26 Prickett JD, Robinson DR, Steinberg AD { 1981) Dietary enrichment with the polyunsaturated fatty acid eicosapentaenoic acid prevents proteinuria and prolongs survival in NZB x NZW mice. *J Clin Invest* 68: 556–559

27 Kelley VE, Ferretti A, Izui S, Strom TB (1985) A fish oil diet rich in eicosapentaenoic acid reduces cyclooxygenase metabolites and suppresses lupus in MRL/lpr mice. *J Immunol* 134: 1914–1919

28 Leslie CA, Gonnerman WA, Ullman MD, Hayes KC, Franzblau C, Cathcart ES (1985) Dietary fish oil modulates macrophage fatty acids and decreases arthritis susceptibility in mice. *J Exp Med* 162: 1336–1349

29 Sperling RI (1995) Eicosanoids in rheumatoid arthritis. *Rheumat Dis Clin N Amer* 21: 741–758

30 De Luca P, Rothman D, Zurier RB (1995) Marine and botanic lipids as immunomodulatiry and therapeutic agents in the treatment of rheumatoid arthritis. *Rheumat Dis Clin N Amer* 21: 759–777

31 Cleland LG, Hill CL, James MJ (1995) Diet and arthritis. *Baillière's Clin Rheumatol* 9: 771–785

32 Kremer JM (1996) Effects of modulation of inflammatory and immune parameters with rheumatic and inflammatory disease receiving dietary supplementation of *n*-3 and *n*-6 fatty acids. *Lipids* 31: S243–S247

33 James MJ, Cleland LG (1997) Dietary *n*-3 fatty acids and therapy for rheumatoid arthritis. *Semin Arthritis Rheum* 27: 85–97

34 Gürsel T, Firat S, Ercan ZS (1997) Increased serum leukotriene B4 level in the active stage of rheumatoid arthritis in children. *Prostaglandins, Leukotrienes and Essential Fatty Acids* 56: 205–207

35 Robinson DR, Tashjian AH, Levine L (1975) Prostaglandin E2 induced bone resorption by rheumatoid synovia. A model of bone destruction in RA. *J Clin Invest* 56: 1181–1187

36 Rïstimaki A, Garfinkel S, Wessendorf J, Masiag T, Hla T (1994) Induction of cyclooxygenase-2 by interleukin-1α. Evidence for post-transcriptional regulation. *J Biol Chem* 269: 11769–11775

37 Mehindate K, Al-Daccak R, Dayer JM (1995) Superantigen-induced collagenase gene expression in human IFN-γ-treated fibroblast-like synoviocytes involves prostaglandin E2. *J Immunol* 155: 3570–3577

38 Sperling RI, Weinblatt M, Robin JL, Ravalese J, Hoover RL, House F, Coblyn JS, Fraser PA, Spur BW, Robinson DR, Lewis RA, Austin KF (1987) Effect of dietary supplementation with marine fish oil on leucocyte mediator generation and function in rheumatoid arthritis. *Arthritis Rheum* 30: 988

39 Espersen GT, Grunnet N, Lervang HH et al (1992) Decreased interleukin-1β levels in plasma from rheumatoid arthritis after dietary supplementation with *n*-3 polyunsaturated fatty acids. *Clin Rheum* 11: 393–395

40 Endres S (1996) *n*-3 polyunsaturated fatty acids and human cytokine synthesis. *Lipids* 31: S239–242

41 Forest C, Franckhauser S, Glorian M, Antras-Ferry J, Robin D, Robin D (1997) Regulation of gene transcription by fatty acids, fibrates and prostaglandins: the phosphoenolpyruvate carboxykinase gene as a modal. *Prostaglandins, Leukotrienes and Essential Fatty Acids* 57: 47–56

42 Nunez EA (1997) Fatty acids involved in signal cross-talk between cell membrane and nucleus. *Prostaglandins, Leukotrienes and Essential Fatty Acids* 57: 429–434

43 Shapiro JA, Koepsell TD, Voigt LF, Dugowson CE, Kestin M, Nelson JL (1996) Diet and rheumatoid arthritis: a possible protective effect of fish consumption. *Epidemiology* 7: 256–263

44 Kremer JM, Bigaouette J (1996) Nutritient intake of patients with rheumatoid arthritis is deficient in pyridoxine, zinc, copper and magnesium. *J Rheumatol* 23: 990–994

45 Fortin PR, Lew RA, Liang MH, Wright EA, Beckett LA, Chalmers TC, Sperling RI (1995) Validation of a meta-analysis: the effects of fish oil in rheumatoid arthritis. *J Clin Epidemiol* 48: 1379–1390

46 Belch JJ, Ansel D, Madhok et al (1988) Effects of altering dietary essential fatty acids on requirements for non-steroidal antiinflammarory drugs in patients with rheumatoid arthritis: a double-blind placebo controlled study. *Ann Rheumat Dis* 47: 96–104

47 Tulleken JE (1991) *Long chain omega-3 polyunsaturated fatty acids in rheumatoid arthritis*. Rijksuniversiteit Groningen, Thesis

48 Belluzzi A, Brignola C, Campieri M, Pera A, Bosch S, Miglioli M (1996) Effect of enteric-coated fish-oil preparation on relapses in Crohn's disease. *N Engl J Med* 334: 1557–1560

49 Caughey GE, Mantzioris E, Gibson RA, Cleland LG, James MJ (1996) The effect on human tumor necrosis factor α and interleukin-1β production of diets enriched in *n*-3 fatty acids from vegetable oil or fish oil. *Am J Clin Nutr* 63: 116–122

50 Nettleton JA (1991) Omega-3 Fatty acids: comparison of plant and seafood sources in human nutrition. *J Am Diet Assoc* 91: 331–337

51 Cleland LG, James MJ (1997) Rheumatoid arthritis and balance of dietary *n*-6 and *n*-3 essential fatty acids. *Brit J Rheumatol* 36: 513–515

52 Boers M, Verhoeven AC, Markusse HM, van de Laar MA, Westhovens R, van Denderen JC, van Zeben D, Dijkmans BA, Peeters AJ, Jacobs P, van den Brink HR, Schouten HJ, van der Heijde DM, Boonen A, van der Linden S (1997) Randomised comparison of combined step-down prednisolone, methotrexate and sulphasalazine with sulphasalazine alone in early rheumatoid arthritis. *Lancet* 2: 309–318

n-3 Polyunsaturated fatty acids in the treatment of patients with IgA nephropathy

Joseph P. Grande[1] and James V. Donadio[2]

[1]Division of Anatomic Pathology, Department of Laboratory Medicine and Pathology and Division of Nephrology, Department of Internal Medicine, Mayo Clinic, 200 First Street SW, Rochester, MN 55905, USA; [2]Chair, Emeritus; Division of Nephrology, Department of Internal Medicine, Mayo Clinic, 200 First Street SW, Rochester, MN 55905, USA

Introduction

First described in 1968 by Berger and Hinglais [1], immunoglobulin A nephropathy (IgAN) is now recognized as the most commonly encountered primary glomerulonephritis worldwide [2–4]. IgAN is an immune complex-mediated glomerular disease defined morphologically by the constant presence of predominant or codominant mesangial deposits of IgA accompanied by a variety of proliferative and/or sclerosing histopathologic lesions [5]. IgAN is characterized by a highly variable clinical course with many patients developing a chronic, slowly progressive decline in renal function over 10–20 years [6–12]. Due to a poorly understood pathogenesis, and because of the variability of the disease, it has been difficult to determine optimal therapy for patients with IgAN [13]. To provide rationale for novel therapeutic agents capable of preserving renal function, there has been active interest in elucidating histopathologic features that confer a high risk of disease progression in patients with IgAN.

Pathophysiology of IgAN

A renal biopsy, demonstrating glomerular deposition of IgA, is essential for the diagnosis of IgAN. Light microscopic alterations are variable and may include minimal light microscopic alterations, mesangial proliferation, focal or diffuse endocapillary proliferation, extracapillary proliferation, and prominent segmental or global glomerulosclerosis. By immunofluorescence, IgA is the predominant or codominant immune reactant; variable deposition of IgG or IgM may also be noted. The deposits are predominantly within mesangial regions of all glomeruli. Ultrastructural evaluation confirms the light microscopic and immunofluorescence findings.

Medicinal Fatty Acids in Inflammation, edited by J.M. Kremer

Current evidence supports the hypothesis that IgAN is a systemic immune complex disease resulting from poorly controlled mucosal immune responses to environmental antigens [14]. However, in human IgAN, no antigen has been definitively identified. IgAN recurs in renal allografts [15]. When a cadaveric kidney containing IgA deposits is transplanted into a recipient with no history of IgAN, the deposits in the grafted kidney rapidly disappear [16]. These observations suggest that renal IgA deposition is due to systemic, humoral factors in patients with IgAN. It is not clear whether immune complexes are deposited in the mesangium from the circulation or by *in situ* formation of IgA antibodies to "planted" antigens absorbed from either the digestive or respiratory tracts [17]. Both viral and bacterial infections, especially of the respiratory tract, have been implicated as possible sources of antigen in IgAN as well as in the systemic disorder Henoch-Schönlein purpura, considered by some to be an extension of the primary kidney disease [18, 19], which might lead to the formation of IgA-containing immune complexes within the kidney. An immunization process is more likely to occur in individuals who have either altered helper-suppressor T-cell function or impaired macrophage phagocytic activity [20]. Further determinants of immune complex formation relate to anionic antigen localization involving interaction between non-immune cationic proteins derived from inflammatory cells and platelets and glomerular anionic sites [21].

Deposition of the complement component C3 is frequently observed within renal biopsy specimens of symptomatic patients with IgAN and may play a role in renal dysfunction [14]. Glomerular deposition of C3 promotes hematuria in animal models [22]; complement depletion with cobra venom factor, which depletes C3 and distal components of the complement cascade by generating a homologue of the alternative pathway convertase prevents hematuria in murine IgA models [23, 24]. Cultured rat mesangial cells and glomerular epithelial cells bear receptors similar to CR1; binding of activated C3 to CR1 stimulates eicosanoid synthesis [25, 26]. Glomerular cells produce a wide variety of inflammatory mediators, including eicosanoids, acyl glycerol ethers, interleukins, and free radicals in response to immune complexes, complement, phagocytic stimuli, and growth factors/cytokines [25–32].

Macromolecular IgA complexes containing lectins such as gliadin may play an important role in progression of IgAN [33]. Gliadin is capable of binding to both mesangial cells and to IgA at distinct sites facilitating the formation of a macromolecular lattice [17]. Gliadin induces mesangial cell expression of c-myc and c-fos, tumor necrosis factor- (TNF-)α, and interleukin- (IL-)6 mRNA [34]. Gliadin inhibits PGE_2 production and increases TXA_2 production in cultured mesangial cells [33, 34], suggesting that this lectin may act by altering eicosanoid production. Therapeutic efforts directed toward inhibiting effector pathways (eicosanoid biosynthesis, cytokine production, etc.) may be important in preventing the progression of IgAN.

Clinical and histopathologic features of progression in IgAN

In the absence of a well-defined pathogenesis by which IgA deposition leads to progressive renal disease, there has been intense interest in the delineation of clinical and histopathologic features that predict adverse outcome. It is hoped that these markers of progression can be used to determine therapeutic efficacy of agents administered to preserve renal function. By univariate analysis, a large number of clinical features are associated with renal disease progression in patients with IgAN, including hypertension, proteinuria, older age at onset, absence of macroscopic hematuria, and hyperlipidemia [35–37] (Tab. 1).

Histopathologic features associated with renal disease progression in IgAN include overall severity of proliferation [35], cellular crescents [38], glomerular sclerosis, interstitial fibrosis, interstitial inflammation, and vascular sclerosis [35]. Several histopathologic scoring systems have been developed in an attempt to quantify risk of renal disease progression [10, 39, 40]. These features of progression, obtained by univariate analysis, include both sclerotic changes (mesangial or global sclerosis, interstitial fibrosis, tubular atrophy) and active changes (glomerular proliferation, interstitial inflammation) [36, 37]. Many of the histopathologic markers – glomerular sclerosis, interstitial fibrosis, vascular sclerosis – are indicators of longstanding renal disease or of previous renal damage. It has been postulated that hemodynamic alterations may be important in the progression of these forms of injury in IgAN [41]. In a series of 73 patients who underwent repeat biopsies, progression of renal disease was associated with progressive scarring in the interstitial and vascular compartments of the kidney but not the glomerular compartment [42].

Several studies have utilized multivariate analysis to identify clinical and histopathologic features that independently predict adverse outcome in patients with IgAN [11, 12, 43, 44]. In a recent study of 148 patients with IgAN, total glomerular score, a semiquantitative index of glomerular proliferation, inflammation, and extracellular matrix deposition, emerged as an independent predictor of renal failure [11]. Clinical characteristics that were strong predictors of renal failure included elevated serum creatinine concentration, hypertension, and proteinuria at

Table 1 - Clinical and histopathologic features of progression in IgAN

Clinical features	Inflammatory lesions	Sclerosing lesions
Proteinuria	Glomerular proliferation	Segmental glomerulosclerosis
Hypertension	Cellular crescent formation	Global glomerulosclerosis
Hyperlipidemia	Interstitial inflammation	Interstitial fibrosis
		Tubular atrophy
		Vascular sclerosis

diagnosis [11]. There is evidence that *n*-3 polyunsaturated fatty acids (PUFAs) may prevent the development of several of these features of progressive disease (Tab. 1).

Although glomerular, interstitial, and vascular sclerosis are strong predictors of adverse outcome in patients with IgAN, these features likely reflect severe renal insufficiency at the time of diagnostic biopsy. For this reason, there has been interest in defining prognostic factors in patients presenting with normal renal function at time of biopsy. In a series of 81 patients with normal renal function at time of biopsy, markers of progression (as defined by a decrease in creatinine clearance to less than 60 mL/minute) included proteinuria of greater than 1.0 g/day, hypertension, severe diffuse proliferative glomerulonephritis, diffuse proliferative glomerulonephritis with crescents, and glomerular deposition of fibrinogen-related antigen [45]. In some patients, a rise in blood pressure well before a decrease in renal function during the follow-up period was observed. The extent of proteinuria is arguably the best marker of renal disease progression in patients presenting with normal renal function. The incidence of adverse histopathologic markers (sclerosis, proliferation, interstitial damage, and vascular sclerosis) increases with levels of proteinuria [46, 47]. Since proteinuria is a powerful prognostic marker, even in patients with initially normal renal function, this parameter may be a particularly useful marker in assessing therapeutic efficacy of agents employed to preserve renal function in patients with IgAN.

Potential mechanisms by which *n*-3 PUFAs arrest renal disease progression in IgAN

There are a number of potential mechanisms by which *n*-3 fatty acids can arrest renal disease progression in IgAN. Potential mechanisms include effects on eicosanoid production, cytokine production, matrix deposition, reduction of blood pressure, reduction of proteinuria, or normalization of serum lipid levels. Potential mechanisms by which *n*-3 PUFAs can affect these parameters will be considered.

n-3 PUFAs and eicosanoids

A variety of pathophysiologic reactions, including altered vascular resistance, thrombosis, wound healing, and inflammation, are likely influenced by oxygenated metabolites of arachidonic acid and related to long-chain PUFAs that are collectively termed "eicosanoids" [48, 49]. Eicosanoids important in renal pathophysiology include prostaglandins and leukotrienes, a family of bioactive lipids produced mostly from hydroxylated derivatives of arachidonic acid via the cyclooxygenase and lipoxygenase pathway, respectively. There are several lines of evidence indicating that eicosanoids play an important role in progression of IgAN. In the kidney, thromboxane A_2, generated from 20:4n-6 (arachidonic acid), induces vasoconstriction and mesangial cell contraction [29, 50]. By reverse transcriptase-PCR, thromboxane synthetase was found in 40% of renal biopsy tissues obtained from patients with IgAN, but in 0% of renal tissue isolated from patients without IgAN [51]. IgAN patients with positive thromboxane synthetase mRNA had significantly reduced glomerular filtration rate (GFR) with elevated creatinine and β2 microglobulin levels, compared to IgAN patients that were negative for thromboxane synthetase mRNA. By immunohistochemistry, thromboxane synthetase localized to interstitial infiltrating cells indicating that thromboxanes may be involved in progression of renal inflammation in IgAN. Elevated lipoxygenase pathway products have also been identified in patients with glomerulonephritis, including IgAN [52]. Decreased plasma levels of prostacyclin activity have been described in patients with IgAN [53].

n-3 PUFAs may reduce bioactive eicosanoid production by competing with arachidonic acid as a substrate for cyclooxygenase, by competing with arachidonic acid for the 2-position in membrane phospholipids, or by competing for elongase on desaturase enzymes, thereby decreasing production of arachidonic acid [48]. EPA and DHA undergo biologic transformation to produce trienoic eicosanoids, including prostacyclin (PGI_3), which has vasodilatory and platelet anti-aggregating properties [54], and thromboxane A_3 (TXA_3), which has little vasoconstricting or platelet aggregating properties [55]. EPA is the preferred substrate for products of the lipoxygenase pathway, resulting in the production of an inactive leukotriene B_5 [56, 57]. Leukotriene B_4, a product of arachidonic acid, is a potent chemotactic factor for leukocytes. Therefore, by competing with arachidonic acid, *n*-3 PUFAs may reduce glomerular and interstitial inflammation, reduce mesangial cell contractility, reduce platelet aggregation, and reduce vasoconstriction in response to renal injury. In a murine lupus nephritis model, fish oil reduces leukotriene B_4 production, both by renal parenchymal cells and by circulating mononuclear cells. Decreased leukotriene production is associated with improved renal hemodynamic function and glomerular histology [58]. Fish oil reduces renal thromboxane A_2 generation in adriamycin nephropathy, a model of oxidative renal injury [59].

Growth factor/cytokine production

Glomerular inflammation may reflect the effect of cytokines/growth factors, elaborated in response to glomerular injury, on mesangial cells. Along these lines, elevated γ-interferon (IFNγ) levels are identified in patients with acute exacerbations of IgAN, and blood levels correlate with proliferative activity in renal biopsies as assessed by Ki-67 expression in renal biopsy tissue [60]. Enhanced renal IL-1 gene expression has been observed in immune complex glomerulonephritis [61]. *n*-3 PUFAs inhibit production of the pro-inflammatory cytokines IL-1 and TNF in stimulated peripheral blood mononuclear cells obtained from healthy volunteers [62]. *In vitro*, fish oils inhibit endothelial cell production of a platelet derived growth factor-like substance [29]. DHA is a potent inhibitor of rat uterine stromal cell proliferation [63], an effect that appears to be independent of eicosanoid biosynthesis. In a murine model of lupus, *n*-3 PUFAs markedly decrease renal expression of IL-1β, IL-6, and TNF mRNA [64]. Fish oil also reduces production of other cytokines, including nitric oxide [65]. *n*-3 PUFAs inhibit IL-1-mediated induction of the adhesion molecules E-selectin, ICAM-1, and VCAM-1 in cultured human umbilical cord endothelial cells, suggesting a potential mechanism for the anti-inflammatory properties of fish oil [66]. DHA inhibits IFNγ-induced Ia expression by murine macrophages. This effect appears to be independent of *n*-3 PUFA-mediated pertubations of eicosanoid synthesis [67]. In a preliminary study, *n*-3 PUFAs significantly inhibited mesangial cell proliferation in a rat model of acute mesangial proliferative glomerulonephritis [68]. The mechanism for this effect has not yet been determined.

A characteristic feature of progressive IgAN is glomerular and interstitial deposition of extracellular matrix macromolecules. Transforming growth factor-β (TGF-β) has become recognized as a dominant mediator of extracellular matrix production in progressive renal disease [69–71]. Increased tissue levels of TGF-β are found in patients with progressive IgAN [72]. In a murine model of progressive autoimmune lupus nephritis, amelioration of renal disease by fish oil was associated with significant reduction in renal TGF-β mRNA and protein levels [73]. A potential role for *n*-3 PUFAs in reducing tissue or urine TGF-β levels in patients with IgAN remains to be established.

The mechanism by which *n*-3 PUFAs reduce TGF-β and matrix protein expression has not been defined. However, renal matrix deposition in response to a variety of injurious stimuli, including high glucose, thromboxane A_2, angiotensin II, and endothelin-1, appears to be mediated by protein kinase C-signaled increases in TGF-β1 [74]. Recent studies have demonstrated that fish oil is capable of down-regulating protein kinase C [75] and suppresses mitogen-stimulated increases in diacylglycerol (DAG) activity [76]. The hypothesis that *n*-3 PUFAs inhibit TGF-β1 expression and matrix deposition in patients with IgA nephropathy by inhibiting protein kinase C activation remains to be tested.

Another mechanism by which *n*-3 PUFAs may ameliorate renal injury is by inhibiting the production of reactive oxygen species. Dietary fish oil decreases superoxide generation by human neutrophils, an effect that does not appear to involve the cyclooxygenase pathway [77]. Fish oil and dimethylthiourea (a hydroxyl radical scavenger) synergistically reduces proteinuria and hyperlipidemia in acute adriamycin nephrosis [59]. Renal glutathione content is also increased [59]. Dietary fish oil supplementation reduces superoxide generation in a primate model of ischemia-reperfusion injury [78]. In a murine model of lupus nephritis, *n*-3 lipids increase the expression of antioxidant genes, including catalase, glutathione peroxidase, and superoxide dismutase [64]. Increased antioxidant gene expression by fish oil is associated with a reduction of indices of lipid peroxidation [79]. In cultured cells, similar induction of antioxidant enzymes by *n*-3 PUFAs is observed [80].

Hemodynamic effects

Vascular damage may be modified by the influence of *n*-3 PUFAs on platelet aggregation, plasma lipids, or blood rheology. Fish oil decreases whole blood viscosity and increases red blood cell deformability and flexibility [81]. By inhibiting thromboxane synthesis, EPA inhibits platelet aggregation [82]. PAF-induced aggregation of platelets is reduced following fish oil administration [83]. Fish oil lowers serum triglyceride levels due to decreased hepatic synthesis of very low density lipoprotein (VLDL) [84]. In a study of fish oil in patients with lupus nephritis, fish oil reduced collagen induced platelet aggregation, increased red cell flexibility, and decreased whole blood viscosity [85]. These alterations were associated with a reduction in serum triglycerides by 38% [85]. In humans with primary nephrotic syndrome, fish oil decreased serum triglyceride and cholesterol levels [86]. In several clinical and experimental studies, dietary fish oil supplementation is associated with reduction in blood pressure. Fish oil inhibits the elevation of blood pressure, reduces proteinuria, and reduces the extent of histopathologic damage in stroke-prone spontaneously hypertensive rats [87].

Proteinuria

In models of lupus nephritis, fish oil reduces proteinuria and improves survival [88–90]. These alterations are associated with no change in humoral immunity. In humans with membranous nephropathy and focal segmental glomerulosclerosis, high dose fish oil therapy reduced proteinuria in association with reduction in serum lipid levels [86]. A modest reduction of blood pressure was also noticed, but this did not correlate with proteinuria.

These human and experimental studies have indicated a number of potential mechanisms whereby *n*-3 PUFAs may prevent progression of inflammatory and non-inflammatory forms of renal disease. The relative contribution of decreased serum lipids, reduction in proteinuria, decreased cytokine/growth factor production, or alterations in eicosanoid metabolism need to be considered in the development of a mechanistic hypothesis whereby *n*-3 PUFAs prevent progression of renal disease. With these potential mechanisms in mind, a potential clinical role for *n*-3 PUFAs in IgAN will be considered.

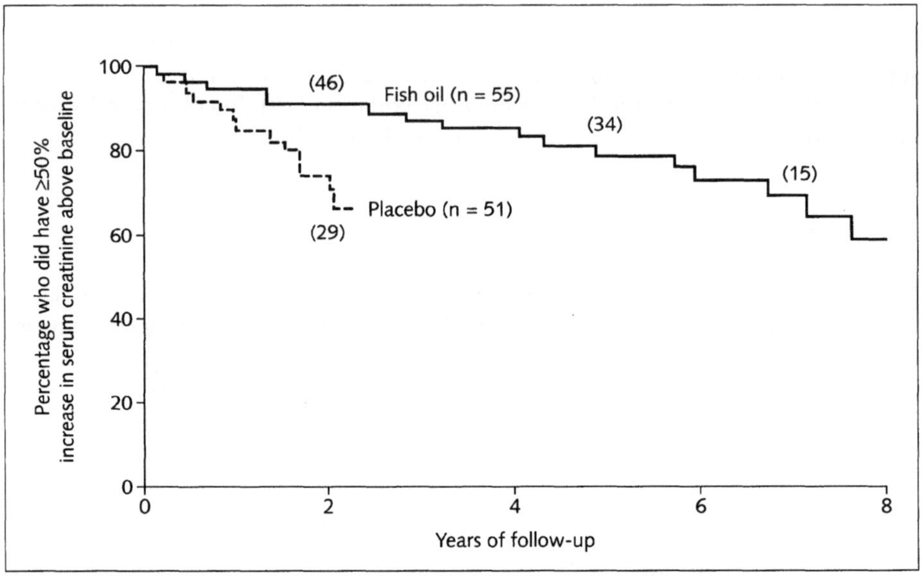

Figure 1
Percentage of patients who did not have ≥50% increase in serum creatinine concentration over baseline (primary end-point) in the long-term follow-up of 55 patients randomized to fish oil. The placebo group was not followed beyond two years because it was no longer a pure control group. The cumulative percent who reached this primary end-point in the fish oil group was 21% at 5 years, compared to 33% at 2 years in the originally assigned placebo group [92]; (n = number of patients at risk).

Clinical studies of fish oil treatment in IgAN

Recent studies have provided support for the hypothesis that fish oil, rich in the *n*-3 PUFAs EPA and DHA, retards renal disease progression in high-risk patients with IgAN [91–93]. It is important to point out, however, that the efficacy of fish oil has been tested in two other clinical trials with negative results [94, 95]. In the largest study – a multicenter, placebo-controlled, randomized trial that included 106 patients – only 6% of patients given a daily dose of fish oil, providing 1.9 g of EPA and 1.4 g of DHA, developed progressive renal failure, whereas 33% of the olive oil placebo group developed progressive renal failure [92]. The study design involved two years of treatment. In extended observations in the 55 patients originally assigned to fish oil, continued treatment with fish oil appears to have reduced the rate at which renal function is lost, consistent with the completed two year trial

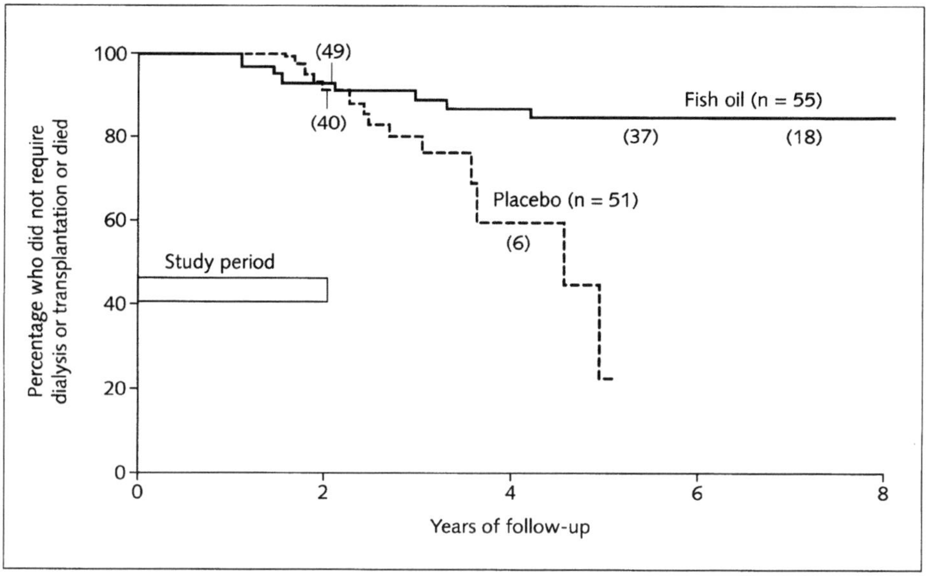

Figure 2
Percentage of patients who did not require dialysis, transplantation, or died. The cumulative percent with end-stage renal disease or death in the fish oil group was 15% at 7 years versus 40% at 4 years in the originally assigned placebo group; (n = number of patients at risk).

[93]. Both the primary end-point defining renal progression, and end-stage renal disease were substantially higher in the placebo group when determined at the conclusion of the clinical trial compared with the longer follow-up of the fish oil-treated group (Figs. 1 and 2).

In three, small sample-sized clinical trials, one study demonstrated a beneficial effect of fish oil [91], while two others did not [94, 95]. Reasons for these discrepant results are not evident but may be related to: Length of follow-up – IgAN is most frequently a slowly progressive disease and long-term studies are required to demonstrate therapeutic efficacy; Blood pressure control – hypertension is an important risk for predicting renal failure; Stage of disease at the time of study – patients with advanced disease evidenced by a serum creatinine concentration above 3 mg/dL developed progressive renal failure despite therapy [96, 97].

With the discrepancy of results in the four published clinical trials testing fish oil, and in an effort to resolve the issue of which is the better treatment for patients at risk of developing progressive renal disease – corticosteroids or *n*-3 PUFAs – two randomized clinical trials are currently underway in the United States [98, 99]. The first trial tests the hypothesis that alternate-day prednisone or daily fish oil will retard the decline in renal function in children and young adults with moderate IgAN [98]. The study design is a randomized, placebo-controlled, multicenter trial conducted by the North American IgA Nephropathy Study Group comprised of both pediatric and internal medicine nephrologists. The second trial tests the hypothesis that an increased amount of *n*-3 PUFAs will influence clearly progressive IgAN [99]. The design is an open-label, comparative dose study using a highly concentrated form of *n*-3 PUFAs (Omacor™) and is being conducted by our collaborative group.

Optimal therapy for all patients with IgAN remains to be established. Finding optimal dosing regimens and elucidating a mechanistic hypothesis whereby fish oil prevents progressive renal disease are hampered by our lack of a full understanding of the pathogenetic mechanisms involved in all forms of progressive parenchymal renal disease. Further studies are needed to accurately define the role of fish oil in preventing glomerulosclerosis and interstitial fibrosis, the morphologic hallmark of irreversible renal disease in IgAN.

References

1 Berger J, Hinglais N (1968) Les depots intercapillaires d'IgA – IgG. *J Urol Nephrol* 74: 694–695

2 Sinniah R, Javier AR, Ku G (1981) The pathology of mesangial IgA nephritis with clinical correlation. *Histopathology* 5: 469–490

3 D'Amico G (1987) The commonest glomerulonephritis in the world: IgA nephropathy. *Q J Med* 245: 709–727

4 Julian BA, Waldo B, Rifai A, Mestecky J (1988) IgA nephropathy, the most common glomerulonephritis worldwide. *Am J Med* 84: 129–132

5 Donadio JV, Grande JP (1997) Immunoglobulin A nephropathy: A clinical perspective. *J Am Soc Nephrol* 8: 1324–1332

6 Hood SA, Velosa JA, Holley KE, Donadio JV (1981) IgA-IgG nephropathy: Predictive indices of progressive disease. *Clin Nephrol* 16: 55–62

7 Droz D (1976) Natural history of primary glomerulonephritis with mesangial deposits of IgA. *Contrib Nephrol* 2: 150–157

8 Droz D, Kramar A, Nawar T, Noel LH (1984) Primary IgA nephropathy: Prognostic factors. *Contrib Nephrol* 40: 202–207

9 Schmekel B, Svalander C, Bucht H, Westberg NG (1981) Mesangial IgA glomerulonephritis in adults. *Acta Med Scand* 210: 363–372

10 Lee S-MK, Rao VM, Franklin WA, Schiffer MS, Aronson AJ, Spargo BH, Katz AI (1982) IgA nephropathy: Morphologic predictors of progressive renal disease. *Hum Pathol* 13: 314–322

11 Radford MG, Donadio JV, Bergstralh EJ, Grande JP (1997) Predicting renal outcome in IgA nephropathy. *J Am Soc Nephrol* 8: 199–207

12 Ibels LS, Gyory AZ (1994) IgA nephropathy: Analysis of the natural history, important factors in the progression of renal disease, and a review of the literature. *Medicine* 73: 79–102

13 Feehally J (1994) Strategies for the management of IgA nephropathy. In: *Annual Yearbook of Nephrology, Dialysis and Transplantation.* Oxford University Press, Oxford, UK, 23–29.

14 Emancipator SN, Lamm ME (1989) IgA nephropathy: Pathogenesis of the most common form of glomerulonephritis. *Lab Invest* 60: 168–183

15 Frohnert PP, Donadio JV, Velosa JA, Holley KE, Sterioff S (1997) The fate of renal transplants in patients with IgA nephropathy. *Clin Transplant* 11: 127–133

16 Berger J (1983) Studies on mesangial IgA glomerulonephritis. *Kidney Int* 24: 408

17 Coppo R, Emancipator S (1994) Pathogenesis of IgA nephropathy: Established observations, new insights and perspectives in treatment. *J Nephrol* 7: 5–15

18 McCoy RC, Abramowsky CR, Tisher CC (1974) IgA nephropathy. *Am J Pathol* 76: 123–144

19 Silva FG (1988) Overview of pediatric nephropathology. *Kidney Int* 33: 1016–1032

20 Rodicio JL (1984) Idiopathic IgA nephropathy. *Kidney Int* 25: 717–729

21 Couser WG (1985) Mechanisms of glomerular injury in immune complex disease. *Kidney Int* 28: 569–583

22 Emancipator SN, Lamm ME (1987) The role of IgG, IgM, and C3 in experimental murine IgA nephropathy. *Semin Nephrol* 7: 286–288

23 Emancipator SN, Ovary Z, Lamm ME (1987) The role of mesangial complement in the hematuria of experimental IgA nephropathy. *Lab Invest* 57: 269–276

24 Cochrane CG, MullerEberhard HJ, Aikin BS (1970) Depletion of plasma complement *in vivo* by a protein of cobra venom: Its effect on various immunologic reactions. *J Immunol* 105: 55–69

25 Habib RB, Stork JE, Emancipator SN (1987) Complement on immune complexes (IC) or zymosan (Z) stimulates prostaglandin (PG) E2 synthesis by glomeruli and cultured glomerular epithelial cells. *Fed Proc* 46: 1329

26 Stork JE, Dunn MJ, Emancipator SN (1985) Identification of complement receptor (CR1) on rat glomerular cells: Effects of complement on prostaglandin synthesis. *Clin Res* 33: 589

27 Sedor JR, Carey SW, Emancipator SN (1987) Immune complexes bind to cultured rat glomerular mesangial cells to stimulate superoxide release. *J Immunol* 138 (11): 3751–3757

28 Lovett DH, Szamel M, Ryan JL, Sterzel RB, Gemsa D, Resch K (1986) Interleukin 1 and the glomerular mesangium. I. Purification and characterization of a mesangial cell-derived auto-growth factor. *J Immunol* 136: 3700–3705

29 Scharschmidt LA, Lianos E, Dunn MJ (1983) Arachidonate metabolites and the control of glomerular function. *Fed Proc* 42: 3058–3063

30 Werber HI, Emancipator SN, Tykocinski ML, Sedor JR (1987) The interleukin 1 gene is expressed by rat glomerular mesangial cells and is augmented in immune complex glomerulonephritis. *J Immunol* 138: 3207–3212
31 Schlondorff D, Satriano JA, Hagege J, Perez J, Baud L (1984) Effect of platelet-activating factor and serum-treated zymosan on prostaglandin E2 synthesis, arachidonic acid release, and contraction of cultured rat mesangial cells. *J Clin Invest* 73: 1227–1231
32 Baud L, Hagege J, Sraer J, Rondeau E, Perez J, Ardaillou R (1983) Reactive oxygen production by cultured rat glomerular mesangial cells during phagocytosis is associated with stimulation of lipoxygenase activity. *J Exp Med* 158: 1836–1852
33 Emancipator SN, Rao CS, Amore A, Coppo R, Nedrud JC (1992) Macromolecular properties that promote mesangial binding and mesangiopathic nephritis. *J Am Soc Nephrol* 2: S149–S158
34 Amore A, Cavallo F, Bocchietto E, Bussolino F, Gianoglio B, Peruzzi L, Porcellini MG, Coppo R (1993) Cytokine mRNA expression by cultured rat mesangial cells after contact with environmental lectins. *Kidney Int* 43: S41–S46
35 Mustonen J, Pasternack A, Helin H, Nikkila M (1985) Clinicopathologic correlations in a series of 143 patients with IgA glomerulonephritis. *Am J Nephrol* 5: 150–157
36 Kobayashi Y, Tateno S, Hiki Y, Shigematsu H (1983) IgA nephropathy: Prognostic significance of proteinuria and histological alterations. *Nephron* 34: 146–153
37 Velo M, Lozano L, Egido J, Gutierrez-Millet V, Hernando L (1987) Natural history of IgA nephropathy in patients followed up for more than ten years in Spain. *Semin Nephrol* 7: 346–350
38 Abe T, Kida H, Yoshimura M et al (1986) Participation of extracapillary lesions (ECL) in progression of IgA nephropathy. *Clin Nephrol* 25: 37–41
39 Donadio JV, Bergstralh EJ, Offord KP, Holley KE, Spencer DC (1994) Clinical and histopathologic associations with impaired renal function in IgA nephropathy. *Clin Nephrol* 41: 65–71
40 Haas M (1997) Histologic subclassification of IgA nephropathy: A clinicopathologic study of 244 cases. *Am J Kidney Dis* 29: 829–842
41 Woodroffe AJ, Bannister KM, Bellon MS, Hale GM, Clarkson AR (1987) Do local hemodynamic alterations mediate injury in IgA nephropathy? *Semin Nephrol* 7: 341–343
42 Alamartine E, Sabatier JC, Berthoux FC (1990) Comparison of pathological lesions on repeated renal biopsies in 73 patients with primary IgA glomerulonephritis: Value of quantitative scoring and approach to final prognosis. *Clin Nephrol* 34: 45–51
43 D'Amico G, Minetti L, Ponticelli C, Fellin G, Ferrario F, Di Belgioioso GB, Imbasciati E, Ragni A, Bertoli S, Fogazzi G et al (1986) Prognostic indicators in idiopathic IgA mesangial nephropathy. *Q J Med* 228: 363–378
44 Alamartine E, Sabatier J-C, Guerin C, Berliet J-M, Berthoux F (1991) Prognostic factors in mesangial IgA glomerulonephritis: An extensive study with univariate and multivariate analysis. *Am J Kidney Dis* 18: 12–19

45 Chida Y, Tomura S, Takeuchi J (1985) Renal survival rate of IgA nephropathy. *Nephron* 40: 189–194

46 Gallo GR, Katafuchi R, Neelakantappa K, Baldwin DS (1988) Prognostic pathologic markers in IgA nephropathy. *Am J Kidney Dis* 12: 362–365

47 Neelakantappa K, Gallo GR, Baldwin DS (1987) Proteinuria in IgA nephropathy. *Semin Nephrol* 7: 344–345

48 Donadio JV (1991) Omega-3 polyunsaturated fatty acids: A potential new treatment of immune renal disease. *Mayo Clin Proc* 66: 1018–1028

49 Donadio JV (1993) An overview of *n*-3 fatty acids in clinical renal diseases. In: R De Caterina, S Endres, SD Kristensen, EB Schmidt (eds): *Current topics in cardiovascular disease.* 1st ed. Bi & Gi Publishers, Verona, Italy, 123–132

50 Sakr HM, Dunham EW (1982) Mechanism of arachidonic acid-induced vasoconstriction in the intact rat kidney: possible involvement of thromboxane A2. *J Pharmacol Exp Ther* 221: 614–622

51 Endoh M, Kashem A, Yamauchi F, Yano N, Nomoto Y, Sakai H, Kurokawa K (1997) Expression of thromboxane synthase in kidney tissues from patients with IgA nephropathy. *Clin Nephrol* 47: 168–175

52 Rifai A, Sakai H, Yagame M (1993) Expression of 5-lipoxygenase and 5-lipoxygenase activation protein in glomerulonephritis. *Kidney Int* 39: S95–S99

53 Turi S, Nagy J, Haszon I, Havass Z, Nemeth M, Bereczki C (1988) Disturbances of lipoprotein and PGI2 metabolism in IgA nephropathy and Henoch-Schönlein purpura. *Contrib Nephrol* 67: 37–43

54 Fischer S, Weber PC (1984) Prostaglandin I3 is formed *in vivo* in man after dietary eicosapentaenoic acid. *Nature* 307: 165–168

55 Fischer S, Weber PC (1983) Thromboxane A3 (TXA3) is formed in human platelets after dietary eicosapentaenoic acid (C20: 5 omega 3). *Biochem Biophys Res Commun* 116: 1091–1099

56 Lee TH, Mencia-Huerta J-M, Corey EJ, Lewis RA, Austen KF (1984) Effects of exogenous arachidonic, eicosapentaenoic, and docosahexaenoic acids on the generation of 5-lipoxygenase pathway products by ionophore-activated human neutrophils. *J Clin Invest* 74: 1922–1933

57 Weaver BJ, Holub BJ (1988) Health effects and metabolism of dietary eicosapentaenoic acid. *Prog Food Nutr Sci* 12: 111–150

58 Spurney RF, Ruiz P, Albrightson CR, Pisetsky DS, Coffman TM (1994) Fish oil feeding modulates leukotriene production in murine lupus nephritis. *Prostaglandins* 48: 331–348

59 Milner LS, Wei S, Kazakoff P, Watkins L, Houser MT (1994) Synergistic effects of fish oil diet and dimethylthiourea in acute adriamycin nephrosis. *Am J Med Sci* 308: 266–270

60 Yokoyama H, Takaeda M, Wada T, Ogi M, Tomosugi N, Takabatake T, Abe T, Yoshimura M, Kida H, Kobayashi K (1992) Intraglomerular expression of MHC class

II and Ki-67 antigens and serum gamma-interferon levels in IgA nephropathy. *Nephron* 62: 169–175
61 Bruno S, Crissman HA, Bauer KD, Darzynkiewicz Z (1991) Changes in cell nuclei during S phase: Progressive chromatin condensation and altered expression of the proliferation associated nuclear proteins Ki-67, cyclin (PCNA), p105, and p34. *Exp Cell Res* 196: 99–106
62 Endres S, Ghorbani R, Kelley VE, Georgilis K, Lonnemann G, van der Meer JWM, Cannon JG, Rogers TS, Klempner MS, Weber PC et al (1989) The effect of dietary supplementation with *n*-3 polyunsaturated fatty acids on the synthesis of interleukin-1 and tumor necrosis factor by mononuclear cells. *N Engl J Med*; 320: 265–271
63 Tessier C, Fayard J-M, Cohen H, Pageaux J-F, Lagarde M, Laugier C (1995) Docosahexaenoic acid is a potent inhibitor of rat uterine stromal cell proliferation. *Biochem Biophys Res Commun* 207: 1015–1021
64 Chandrasekar B, Fernandes G (1994) Decreased pro-inflammatory cytokines and increased antioxidant enzyme gene expression by ω-3 lipids in murine lupus nephritis. *Biochem Biophys Res Comm* 200: 893–898
65 Boutard V, Fouqueray B, Philippe C, Perez J, Baud L (1994) Fish oil supplementation and essential fatty acid deficiency reduce nitric oxide synthesis by rat macrophages. *Kidney Int* 46: 1280–1286
66 Eddy AA, Giachelli CM (1995) Renal expression of genes that promote interstitial inflammation and fibrosis in rats with protein-overload proteinuria. *Kidney Int* 47: 1546–1557
67 Khair-El-Din TA, Sicher SC, Vazquez MA, Wright WJ, Lu CY (1995) Docosahexaenoic acid, a major constituent of fetal serum and fish oil diets, inhibits IFNγ-induced Ia-expression by murine macrophages *in vitro*. *J Immunol* 154: 1296–1306
68 Grande JP, Walker HJ, Donadio JV, Dousa TP (1997) Omega-3 fatty acids inhibit mesangial cell proliferation in proliferative glomerulonephritis. *J Invest Med* 45: 279A
69 Border WA, Noble NA, Ketteler M (1995) TGF-beta: A cytokine mediator of glomerulosclerosis and a target for therapeutic intervention. *Kidney Int* 47: S59–S61
70 Grande JP (1997) Role of transforming growth factor-beta in tissue injury and repair. *Proc Soc Exp Biol Med* 214: 27–40
71 Grande JP, Melder DC, Zinsmeister AR (1997) Modulation of collagen gene expression by cytokines: Stimulatory effect of transforming growth factor-β1, with divergent effects of epidermal growth factor and tumor necrosis factor-α on collagen type I and collagen type IV. *J Lab Clin Med* 130: 476–486
72 Niemir ZI, Stein H, Noronha IL, Kruger C, Andrassy K, Ritz E, Waldherr R (1995) PDGF and TGF-beta contribute to the natural course of human IgA glomerulonephritis. *Kidney Int* 48: 1530–1541
73 Chandrasekar B, Troyer DA, Venkatraman JT, Fernandes G (1995) Dietary omega-3 lipids delay the onset and progression of autoimmune lupus nephritis by inhibiting transforming growth factor β mRNA and protein expression. *J Autoimmun* 8: 381–393

74 Studer RK, Craven PA, DeRubertis FR (1997) Antioxidant inhibition of protein kinase C-signaled increases in transforming growth factor-beta in mesangial cells. *Metabolism* 46(8): 918–925

75 Nakamura T, Takahashi T, Fukui M et al (1995) Enalapril attenuates increased gene expression of extracellular matrix components in diabetic rats. *J Am Soc Nephrol* 5: 1492–1497

76 Thomazy V, Fesus L (1989) Differential expression of tissue transglutaminase in human cells: An immunohistochemical study. *Cell Tissue Res* 255: 215–224

77 Chini EN, Chini CCS, Bollinger C, Jougasaki M, Grande JP, Burnett JC, Dousa TP (1997) Cytoprotective effects of adrenomedullin in glomerular cell injury: Central role of cAMP signaling pathway. *Kidney Int* 52: 917–925

78 Eddy AA (1994) Experimental insights into the tubulointerstitial disease accompanying primary glomerular lesions. *J Am Soc Nephrol* 5: 1273–1287

79 Venkatraman JT, Chandrasekar B, Kim JD, Fernandes G (1994) Effects of *n*-3 and *n*-6 fatty acids on the activities and expression of hepatic antioxidant enzymes in autoimmune-prone NZBxNZW F1 mice. *Lipids* 29: 561–568

80 Morita Y, Nomura A, Yuzawa Y, Nishikawa K, Hotta N, Shimizu F, Matsuo S (1997) The role of complement in the pathogenesis of tubulointerstitial lesions in rat mesangial proliferative glomerulonephritis. *J Am Soc Nephrol* 8: 1363–1372

81 Cartwright IJ, Pockley AG, Galloway JH, Greaves M, Preston FE (1985) The effects of dietary omega-3 polyunsaturated fatty acids on erythrocyte membrane phospholipids, erythrocyte deformability, and blood viscosity in healthy volunteers. *Atherosclerosis* 55: 267–281

82 Driss F, Vericel E, Lagarde M, Dechavanne M, Darcet P (1984) Inhibition of platelet aggregation and thromboxane synthesis after intake of small amount of eicosapentaenoic acid. *Thromb Res* 36: 389–396

83 Skeaff CM, Holub BJ (1988) The effect of fish oil consumption on platelet aggregation responses in washed human platelet suspensions. *Thromb Res* 51: 105–115

84 Phillipson BE, Rothrock DW, Connor WE, Harris WS, Illingworth DR (1985) Reduction of plasma lipids, lipoproteins, and apoproteins by dietary fish oils in patients with hypertriglyceridemia. *N Engl J Med* 312: 1210–1216

85 Clark WF, Parbtani A, Huff MW, Reid B, Holub BJ, Falardeau P (1989) Omega-3 fatty acid dietary supplementation in systemic lupus erythematosus. *Kidney Int* 36: 653–660

86 De Caterina R, Caprioli R, Giannessi D, Sicari R, Galli C, Lazzerini G, Bernini W, Carr L, Rindi P (1993) *n*-3 fatty acids reduce proteinuria in patients with chronic glomerular disease. *Kidney Int* 44: 843–850

87 Hobbs LM, Rayner TE, Howe PRC (1996) Dietary fish oil prevents the development of renal damage in salt-loaded stroke-prone spontaneously hypertensive rats. *Clin Exp Pharmacol Physiol* 23: 508–513

88 Prickett JD, Robinson DR, Steinberg AD (1981) Dietary enrichment with the polyunsaturated fatty acid eicosapentaenoic acid prevents proteinuria and prolongs survival in NZB X NZW F1 mice. *J Clin Invest* 68: 556–559

89 Prickett JD, Robinson DR, Steinberg AD (1983) Effects of dietary enrichment with eicosapentaenoic acid upon autoimmune nephritis in female NZB x NZW/F1 mice. *Arthritis Rheum* 26: 133–139
90 Robinson DR, Prickett JD, Makoul GT, Steinberg AD, Colvin RB (1986) Dietary fish oil reduces progression of established renal disease in (NZB x NZW)F1 mice and delays renal disease in BXSB and MRL/1 strains. *Arthritis Rheum* 29: 539–546
91 Hamazaki T, Tateno S, Shishido H (1984) Eicosapentaenoic acid and IgA nephropathy. *Lancet* 1: 1017–1018
92 Donadio JV, Bergstralh EJ, Offord KP, Spencer DC, Holley KE (1994) A controlled trial of fish oil in IgA nephropathy. *N Engl J Med* 331: 1194–1199
93 Donadio JV, Dart RA, Grande JP, Bergstralh EJ, Spencer DC (1997) Long-term treatment with fish oil reduces renal progression in patients with IgA nephropathy (IgAN). *J Am Soc Nephrol* 8: 85A
94 Bennett WM, Walker RG, Kincaid-Smith P (1989) Treatment of IgA nephropathy with eicosapentaenoic acid (EPA): A two year prospective trial. *Clin Nephrol* 31: 128–131
95 Pettersson EE, Rekola S, Berglund L, Sundqvist KG, Angelin B, Diczfalusy U, Björkhem I, Bergström J (1994) Treatment of IgA nephropathy with omega-3-polyunsaturated fatty acids: A prospective, double-blind, randomized study. *Clin Nephrol* 41: 183–190
96 Cheng IKP, Chan PCK, Chan MK (1990) The effect of fish-oil dietary supplement on the progression of mesangial IgA glomerulonephritis. *Nephrol Dial Transplant* 5: 241– 246
97 Fung SM, Ferrill MJ, Norton LL (1997) Fish oil therapy in IgA nephropathy. *Ann Pharmacother* 31: 112–115
98 Hogg RJ (1995) A randomized, placebo-controlled, multicenter trial evaluating alternate-day prednisone and fish oil supplements in young patients with IgA nephropathy. *Am J Kidney Dis* 26: 792–796
99 Donadio JV, Bergstralh EJ, Offord KP, Grande JP, Larson TS, Spencer DC. A prospective comparative study of two doses of Omacor™ in the treatment of patients with IgA nephropathy. *In progress*

Subject index

PIR
Progress in Inflammation Research

Miossec P., Hôpital Edouard Herriot, Lyon, France / **van den Berg W.B.,** University Hospital Nijmegen, Netherlands / **Firestein G.S.,** UCSD, La Jolla, USA

T Cells in Arthritis

1998. 238 pages. Hardcover
ISBN 3-7643-5853-X

Rheumatoid arthritis (RA) is the most common and most severe form of inflammatory arthritis. The pathogenesis of RA has been the subject of intense research for several decades. The prevailing hypotheses have changed over the years, and have attempted to incorporate the most recent data. Although T cells represent an important component of the cells which infiltrate the joint synovium, their contribution at a late stage of the disease remains a matter of debate.

The goal of this book is to outline the major arguments and data suggesting that T cells may, or may not, be central players in the pathogenesis of chronic RA. While each of the editors and authors has his/her own bias (as will be clear by reading the respective chapters), our hope is that the readers will enjoy a complete and balanced view of the critical questions and experiments. This is not just an intellectual exercise since the direction of future therapeutic interventions depends heavily on how one interprets the pathogenesis of RA and the contribution of T cells.

PIR
Progress in Inflammation Research

Redl H. / Schlag G., Ludwig Boltzmann Institute for Experimental and Clinical Traumatology, Vienna, Austria

Cytokines in Severe Sepsis and Septic Shock

1998. Approx. 300 pages. Hardcover
ISBN 3-7643-5877-7
Due in November 1998

This book deals with the central role of cytokines in the generalized inflammatory response of the host as the consequence of severe infection/endotoxin action. International specialists cover several aspects in 20 chapters starting with the agents responsible (endotoxin, superantigens) and recognition during cytokine induction. Further chapters deal with the signal transduction cascade, its modulation due to sex or genetic polymorphism, and the possibilities and problems in detection (including surrogate markers). Major targets of actions are covered in the chapters on coagulation/fibrinolysis, adherence molecules, vasoactive factors, apoptosis and metabolism. As not all actions of cytokines are beneficial, several chapters deal with the prevention of induction, modulation of the cytokine generation or scavenging cytokines including gene therapy approaches. Models are necessary for obtaining pathophysiological information and for testing therapeutic approaches, and thus all chapters deal with experimental models as well as clinical trials. The reasons why these have failed so far are the subject of the final chapter.

Researchers and students of Critical Care Medicine and Biomedicine will find up-to-date reviews and data in this book.

MIX
Papier aus verantwortungsvollen Quellen
Paper from responsible sources
FSC® C105338

If you have any concerns about our products,
you can contact us on
ProductSafety@springernature.com

In case Publisher is established outside the EU,
the EU authorized representative is:
Springer Nature Customer Service Center GmbH
Europaplatz 3, 69115 Heidelberg, Germany

Printed by Libri Plureos GmbH
in Hamburg, Germany